Research, Truth and Authority

Previous books by Gary Rolfe

Closing the Theory–Practice Gap: A New Paradigm for Nursing, Oxford: Butterworth Heinemann (1996)

Expanding Nursing Knowledge: Understanding and Researching Your Own Practice, Oxford: Butterworth Heinemann (1998)

Advanced Nursing Practice (with Paul Fulbrook), Oxford: Butterworth Heinemann (1998)

Research, Truth and Authority

Postmodern Perspectives on Nursing

Gary Rolfe

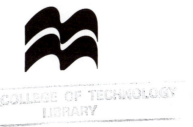

First published 2000 by
MACMILLAN PRESS LTD
Houndmills, Basingstoke, Hampshire RG21 6XS
and London
Companies and representatives throughout the world

ISBN 0–333–77637–2 paperback

A catalogue record for this book is available
from the British Library.

This book is printed on paper suitable for recycling and
made from fully managed and sustained forest sources.

10 9 8 7 6 5 4 3 2 1
09 08 07 06 05 04 03 02 01 00

Editing and origination by
Aardvark Editorial, Mendham, Suffolk

Printed in Malaysia

for my angel
Gabriel

Without Unceasing Practice, nothing can be done.
Practice is Art. If you leave off you are Lost.

William Blake
c. 1820

CONTENTS

Contents

Kathleen Fahy is an academic who is currently co-ordinating the Master of Midwifery course at the University of Southern Queensland. She has practised as a nurse and a midwife, and most recently as a community midwife for marginalized teenage women. Her research methodology is feminist praxis using postmodern theories with emancipatory intent. She has published in the area of midwifery with particular emphasis on power, advocacy and subject position theory.

JoEllen Goetz Koerner has experienced a lifetime career in nursing that has included leadership positions in nursing service (Senior Vice President of Sioux Valley Hospitals and Health System, Sioux Falls, South Dakota), nursing education (Director, Department of Nursing, Freeman College) and nursing regulation (Executive Director of South Dakota Board of Nursing). Her current position as Executive Vice President of Health Care Resources focuses on community health and the weaving of complementary therapies into Western medical protocols for managed care contracts. Nursing's emerging partnership with the public, focused on health and well-being, is a return to our roots as we re-member community.

Claire Parsons qualified and practised as a registered nurse and midwife before commencing an academic career. Since undertaking her doctoral studies in sociology in New Zealand, she has received a number of awards, including the Claude McCarthy fellowship, which she took as a postdoctoral fellow at Harvard, USA. She was recently awarded a Public Health Travelling Fellowship from the National Health and Medical Research Council in Australia. This fellowship allowed her to meet with colleagues in Canada and the USA to assess North American public health nursing research. Claire has published widely in the fields of clinical nursing and public health, for example in cross-cultural health care, women's health and HIV/AIDS. She has also written on ethical and theoretical issues, including those pertaining to research methodology. While Claire maintains both a knowledge and a practice in nursing, she is also currently undertaking research into the changing philosophy of science in medicine, and its impact on health care in the twenty-first century.

Gary Rolfe is principal lecturer in the School of Health and Social Care at the University of Portsmouth, where he teaches and facilitates research and practice development. He has a particular interest in action research and student-centred interdisciplinary education, and has written books on the theory–practice gap, practitioner-based enquiry and advanced nursing practice.

Kim Walker is a nurse whose history as a clinician compels him to orientate his research and scholarship around the cultural politics of nursing and health, particularly in relation to exploring post-positivist methodologies and theoretical frameworks that better engage and interrogate the complexity of contemporary health care. He is currently Director, Professional Services, at the New South Wales College of Nursing and also Senior Research Fellow in the Faculty of Nursing, Midwifery and Health at the University of Technology, Sydney, where he teaches and supervises in the Professional Doctorate and other graduate programmes.

Back to the bedpans
or
Why you should read this book

If the doors of perception were cleansed,
every thing would appear to man as it is, infinite.
For man has closed himself up,
till he sees all things thro' narrow chinks of his cavern.[1]

FROM BEDPANS TO BARTHES

As I write this introduction, in the final months of the twentieth century and almost one hundred and fifty years after Nightingale first went to the Crimea, the opening shots have just been fired in the latest battle in the UK for the heart and soul of nursing. The trigger that sparked off this particular battle was the current shortage of nurses in the NHS, but the battles themselves are always fought over the same territory: whether nursing is (or should be) an academic discipline, and hence whether nurses need to be educated or merely trained.[2]

This time, the debate was triggered by a piece in the British newspaper the *Daily Express* by Melanie Phillips, in which she blamed the current recruitment crisis on the move of nurse training into higher education, where it is being contaminated by 'the nihilistic, politically correct gibberish that has disfigured social sciences'[3] (surely a reference to postmodernism!). This was swiftly followed by Brian Sewell in the *Evening Standard*, who bemoaned the fact that 'nurses now achieve academic levels that far exceed those of many university courses – an appalling waste when applied to their work at the bedpan level',[4] adding that 'one does not need a degree in philosophy to become a gardener'. Nigella Lawson, writing in *The Observer*, denounced Project 2000 as a 'ludicrous proposition',[5] and continued by observing that 'at the moment we treat nursing applicants as if we wanted them to be management executives with the pay rate of Puerto Rican piece workers', with the implication that if we only educated them to the level of piece workers, they could hardly complain about the pay. What all of these writers appear to be suggesting is that rather than provide the pay and conditions that a well-educated professional might expect, the current recruitment crisis would be solved by providing the education that a poorly paid doctor's handmaiden might deserve.

In educational parlance, this approach has euphemistically been termed 'widening the entry gate', and makes the totally unfounded assumption that we might attract more recruits into nursing by making it easier to gain admission. After all, you might not need a degree in philosophy to empty a bedpan, but by the same reasoning, you do not need a GCSE either. Of course, the corollary to this is that if we are not to lose all of these recruits at the first academic hurdle, the educational level of the course must also be lower. Perhaps the answer (and this is not a popular view either inside or outside nursing) is to *raise* the entry gate, so that people who would not normally look twice at nursing as a career might be attracted to it. The corollary to *that*, however, is that we would have to pay them at the same rate as other professionals such as lawyers and doctors. Now, many would, of course, point out that we will always need what the Conservative politician Anne Widdecombe has called the 'bedpan brigade'; who else is going to empty the bedpans? But this attitude arguably displays what Anne Marie Rafferty, writing in the *Guardian* newspaper, has termed 'the old prejudice that intelligence and education cannot blend with care and practicality'.[6] The point is that it is possible to have a brain, an education *and* a degree in philosophy, and still empty a bedpan; after all, most doctors have to do some very messy and unpleasant things, but I would still prefer my GP to have at least one degree.

This view, it would appear, is not shared by many book publishers. Whereas journal editors are, by and large, sympathetic to nursing as an academic discipline, most of the book editors I approached with the manuscript of this text informed me in no uncertain terms that nurses would not buy a book about a theoretical subject such as postmodernism. Nurses, I was told, only buy books that tell them directly, and in simple language, how to do nursing practice.[7] When they do buy theoretical books, they are usually books on nursing theory; when they buy books on biological, sociological or psychological theory, they are books that spell out clear and unambiguous links to nursing practice, since nurses are, apparently, unable to make those links for themselves.

This book does not pretend to do any of these things. It is not the sort of book that a nurse would wish to keep in her pocket for reference purposes in order to pull out and consult whenever she encounters a particularly tricky clinical problem. However, I do not believe that this is the only kind of book that nurses need or want: to claim that nurses only read hands-on practical texts or texts in which the links to practice are spelt out for them is an insult to the intelligence of most nurses as well as displaying Anne Marie Rafferty's 'old prejudice'.

So why read postmodernism? After all, it is not always reader-friendly, and might appear on first sight to have little to say to busy practitioners. But if you can cut through some of the dense language and the (more than) occasional charlatanism, the writing is, at its best, poetic, insightful, amusing and, on occasion, able to bypass the brain and speak directly to the heart.[8] More importantly, however, it has some highly pertinent things to say about life in the twenty-first century, particularly about the relationship between knowledge, power and authority, which is of direct relevance to anyone who has to make decisions based on best evidence (which includes all of us), and also to those of us who have misgivings about where authority is invested in the nursing profession. Reading postmodernism might not make you a better practitioner, but it will hopefully help you to develop a more questioning attitude and make you generally more troublesome to those in the profession who attempt to be authoritarian without being authoritative. In the tradition of postmodernism, I will not attempt to sell it as the answer to all your problems (as what the postmodernists term a 'grand narrative'), but will instead offer you a 'little narrative' in the story of my own 'postmodern turn'.

TAKING THE POSTMODERN TURN

When I first came across postmodernism several years ago, my first instinct was to reject it as academically unsound and irrelevant to nursing, and I secretly hoped that if I ignored it, it would eventually go away. It didn't. As it encroached more and more into my reading and into my life, I decided that I would have to find out what all the fuss was about. However, the task was daunting, not least because every book on the subject that I picked up appeared to say something different. I finally took the plunge with a short book of selections from the writing of Roland Barthes (not strictly speaking a postmodernist), entitled *Image Music Text,*[9] and moved rapidly on to Jacques Derrida, François Lyotard and beyond. In retrospect, my initial dismissal of postmodernism was clearly a defence against having to start from scratch on a vast and daunting new body of literature. Or perhaps I should say 'literatures', since my earlier observation of every book on postmodernism saying something different seemed to be fairly accurate.

Once I started reading, I began to seek out people with whom to discuss my new-found interest, and on speaking to colleagues in nursing and nurse education, I came across three broad responses to the so-called postmodern turn. A few (mostly educationalists) had taken the plunge and found postmodernism to be as fascinating and relevant as I do. A few more had expressed an interest in the subject but did not really know where to start. Most, however, displayed the same initial reaction as I did: they saw it as irrelevant nonsense with nothing to say to nurses, or even to nurse educators. I can, of course, empathize with this attitude, but it nevertheless saddens me, since I now firmly believe that postmodernism is neither nonsense nor irrelevant.

Since my first forays into postmodernism, a number of basic introductory texts have been published, but they all suffer from the same problem, which I alluded to earlier. The problem is this: there is no simple, clear-cut discipline or subject area to which we can give the label 'postmodernism'. There is postmodern architecture, postmodern literature, postmodern philosophy and so on, almost *ad infinitum*. There *are*, of course, threads running through all these postmodernisms, but attempts to articulate or summarize them usually result in banal statements such as 'multiple truths', 'mix and match' or 'anything goes', terms that hardly do justice to the rich tapestry of thought, attitudes and artefacts that constitute postmodernism.

Most successful introductory texts therefore wisely focus on a particular perspective; those which attempt a broader view often leave the reader more confused than enlightened. However, few, if any, of these introductory texts provide a perspective that nurses would find useful or relevant, and those which do are often written in a language that most would find inaccessible.[10]

This book, then, is an unashamed attempt to fill a niche. The book is divided into two parts. The first is a general introduction to the history and some of the key ideas of postmodernism. It is general in that it hardly mentions nursing, but it is nevertheless written for nurses by attempting to focus on the particular aspects of postmodernism that I believe are relevant to nursing. There is thus little about postmodern architecture or cultural theory, but a great deal about postmodern concepts of truth, science and research. Similarly, certain writers, for example Baudrillard and Deleuze, barely get a mention, whereas others, such as Lyotard, Derrida and Rorty, feature extensively. All introductory texts are necessarily selective in the viewpoint they present, but Part I of this book makes a virtue of the fact that it takes an *extremely* selective view, and that it does so in fairly simple language.[11] If it does not help you (in Katz's words) to 'speak and write postmodern', my hope is that it will at least allow you to 'read postmodern'.

Part II is also selective, but it is less focused. Its aim is to collect together a number of papers that present a variety of postmodern perspectives on nursing, in particular on nursing research. The aim here, however, is not a narrow focus, but a broad and eclectic cross-section of the, as yet, very limited literature that has appeared over the past five years or so. All of these papers have previously been published, most (because of their subject matter) in hard-to-obtain journals (journal editors not being *that* sympathetic to academic nursing). They present a broad range of views and opinions that, true to the nature of postmodernism, are often in conflict with each other or even with themselves. They make no claim to be representative of anything or anyone, but offer a convenient and easily accessible repository of postmodern perspectives on nursing and nursing research.

Part II is, however, not just a collection of papers: attempts are made first to locate them in a wider debate about postmodern research, and second to provide some links to the broader (mainly philosophical) literature on postmodernism. Furthermore, the academic level of Part II moves up several notches, building significantly on the basic introductory material from Part I. The reader is therefore encouraged to employ her own personal understanding of postmodernism in her own deconstruction and reconstruction of the text. Finally, in the Epilogue, I explore the role that postmodernism plays in deconstructing the power games of modernist nursing and research, and consider what a postmodernist practice might look like.

My hope, then, is that this book will serve two related purposes. First, I trust that Part I will provide the reader with the knowledge and concepts necessary to take part in an *informed* debate about postmodernism rather than simply to dismiss it as (to quote Melanie Phillips) 'nihilistic, politically correct gibberish'. Second, I hope that it will also equip the reader for a critical reading of the papers that make up Part II and, in particular, to cut through the rather dense writing that is often a feature of postmodern texts. Roland Barthes wrote about the 'reading duty' of the academic,[12] of where it begins and of where it ends. I hope that your reading duty (but also your reading pleasure) extends beyond the obvious nursing and research texts, and that you will find as much of relevance in the vast and diverse literature of postmodernism as I have.

NOTES

1. The epigraphs at the start of each chapter are from the works of William Blake (1757–1827) and are found in *Blake's Poems and Prophesies*, edited

by M. Plowman and published by Dent, London, 1927. Blake was both an empiricist who believed that knowledge could only come to us through our senses, and a mystic who was vehemently opposed to the (then) recently developed method of science as the main (or only) source of that knowledge. For Blake, then, the 'true Man' was 'the Poetic Genius' who 'perceives more than sense (tho' ever so acute) can discover'. The literary critic Ihab Hassan has suggested that, as one of the original critics of the scientific method, Blake might be the first postmodernist, albeit two hundred years before his time. Hassan, I. POSTmodernISM: a paracritical bibliography. In L. Cahoone (ed.) *From Modernism to Postmodernism: An Anthology*, Oxford: Blackwell, 1996, p. 390.

2. This debate extends back at least to Nightingale's time. See, for example, Rafferty, A.M. *The Politics of Nursing Knowledge*, London: Routledge, 1996, Chapter 2.

3. Cited in Payne, D. The knives are out for P2000, *Nursing Times*, 1999, **95**, 4, 14–15.

4. *Ibid.*

5. *Ibid.*

6. Rafferty, A.M. Practice made perfect, *Guardian Higher*, 26 January, 1999, p. iii.

7. I do not believe that *any* book can make you a significantly better practitioner. I wrote at the end of a previous book that 'the only book that will really influence your practice is the one you write yourself', and I still stand by that statement. See Rolfe, G. *Closing the Theory–Practice Gap*, Oxford: Butterworth Heinemann, 1996, p. 236.

8. See, for example, Derrida, J. (1974) *Glas*, Lincoln: University of Nebraska Press, 1990; Derrida, J. (1980) *The Post Card*, Chicago: University of Chicago Press, 1987; Barthes, R. (1973), *The Pleasure of the Text*, New York: Hill & Wang, 1971; Barthes, R. (1975), *Roland Barthes by Roland Barthes*, London: Macmillan, 1995; Barthes, R. (1977), *A Lover's Discourse*, New York: Hill & Wang, 1984. The date in parentheses following the author's name is the year in which the book was first published, being included for historical reasons. The date at the end of the reference is the year of publication of this particular edition.

9. Barthes, R. *Image Music Text*, London: Fontana, 1977.

10. This is not because nurses are any less intelligent or educated than anyone else. The problem is widespread throughout academia, and the interested reader might like to look at Stephen Katz's essay 'How to speak and write postmodern' for a tongue-in-cheek account of the intricacies of postmodern language: Katz, S. How to speak and write postmodern. In W.T. Anderson, *The Fontana Postmodernism Reader*, London: Fontana Press, 1996, pp. 88–91.

11. Although the concepts that it attempts to discuss are far from simple.

12. Barthes, R. (1975) *Roland Barthes by Roland Barthes*, R. Howard (trans.), London: Macmillan, 1995, p. 100.

Part I

TAKING THE POSTMODERN TURN

A fool sees not the same tree a wise man sees.[1]

This is a book about truth, what it is, and how we can come to know it. It is written primarily for nurses and nurse researchers, but it will hopefully also be of interest to social workers, teachers and members of the professions allied to medicine, in fact, all those who are concerned with improving their practice. There is clearly a relationship between truth and good practice: practitioners are urged to base their practice on best evidence of what is effective, and best evidence presumably strives towards what is *truly* most effective for practice. In order to practise effectively, then, nurses and other practitioners in the helping professions require an effective means of identifying and gaining access to the truth.

Nursing and the helping professions are moving ever closer to academia, in terms of both academic qualifications as access to those professions, and an academic base underpinning the way in which they are practised and researched. Furthermore, since there is a clear relationship between academic acceptance and proximity to the hard sciences,[2] most of these professions are currently seeking to improve their scientific status (although some also emphasize the artistic aspect of practice). To aspire to the values of science entails accepting a particular concept of truth, namely that there is something called 'objective truth' that exists 'out there' in the world or, as the argument is sometimes put, that there is an objective reality about which empirical observation can provide 'true' knowledge. The aim of science is thus to uncover this truth (or at least to move ever closer towards it), and the so-called 'scientific method' has been developed over the past four hundred years as the most effective way (some scientists would argue the *only way*) of achieving that aim.

We can see that if good practice relies on effective and reliable access to the truth, and if the truth can best be uncovered through the scientific method, then the scientific method (or what is often referred to as scientific research) is essential to good practice. For many in nursing and the helping professions, evidence-based practice is thus almost synonymous with research-based practice.

Historians and philosophers of science often refer to this attitude towards the concept of truth as 'modernism' or 'the Enlightenment project'. The essence of the Enlightenment project, which is usually considered to have been initiated in the late seventeenth century, is an emphasis on social progress through scientific understanding; that by first understanding how the world functions, we might come to control it for the good of human kind. This ideal of scientific control was later extended to the new disciplines of sociology and psychology, where it came to be known as positivism, and eventually to nursing and the helping professions, where it is sometimes referred to as technical rationality. The basic premise of research-based practice, then, is that by coming to know the truth about how people function physically, psychologically and sociologically, we can exert beneficial control and thereby improve their lot.

There have been a number of challenges to this positivist view during the twentieth century, first from the interpretivist school of sociologists and psychologists who advocated a qualitative approach to data collection and analysis, and latterly from the so-called 'post-positivists' who argued for the relaxation of the rigid correspondence between scientific method and truth. However, these were no more than modifications and adjustments to the scientific paradigm, and, despite some claims to the contrary, never amounted to what Thomas Kuhn termed a paradigm shift.[3]

Arguably the major and most influential challenge to the modernist Enlightenment project has come from the postmodernists, who question the very foundation of modernism, that is, the link between science and truth (and hence the link between research and best practice). From the postmodern perspective, the modernist movement has elevated the scientific method to an unwarranted position as the only means of accessing the truth, and while it might well be effective, that alone does not guarantee its status as gatekeeper to the truth. Indeed, it is argued, circular reasoning is involved: any challenges to the scientific method are usually met with the retort that the findings of scientific research must be true because they produce effective outcomes, and that they produce effective outcomes because they are true.

For the postmodernists, the institution of science is in a position to assert itself as the keeper of the truth because its effectiveness brings with it a great deal of power. Truth, by this account, is whatever those in power say it is, and it therefore shifts along with that power. This, of course, leads to the conclusion that truth cannot be the absolute monolith that the modernists would have us believe, and that it does not exist 'out there' in the world, but is created by social institutions. If, however, concepts of what is true are constantly shifting (or have the potential to shift), the notion of progress is also undermined. Thus, for the postmodernists, the entire Enlightenment project of progress towards truth and social well-being through the methods of science is nothing but an illusion established by those people and institutions with the power to define what truth is. If there is no single, absolute truth, there can be no progress towards that truth, but merely a continual shifting from one equally foundationless value system to another.

In terms of their conceptions of truth, modernism and postmodernism therefore represent the two opposite ends of a spectrum: for the modernists, there is a single absolute truth and a single method (the method of science) for uncovering it; whereas for the postmodernists there are a multitude of 'truths' (which, of course, amounts to the view that there is no absolute truth at all) and a rejection of the scientific method as the only, or even the best, way of uncovering it or them. Indeed, the postmodernists would not even speak of uncovering the truth, since that implies that there is something there waiting to be uncovered; instead, they would see truth as something that is constructed, and there can be as many constructions of the truth as there are people in the world to construct it.

This postmodern challenge to the perceived certainties of modernism is beginning to be felt in nursing and the helping professions, where it tends to result in a rejection of scientific research in favour of an 'anything goes' relativist approach. This, many would argue, can been seen as presenting certain threats to safe practice, and can result in individual practitioners making decisions according to whim rather than best evidence.[4] After all, if there is no absolute truth, one practitioner's notion of good practice is as valid as that of another. Not only does scientific research evidence hold no privileged position over, for example, intuition, or even decisions taken by rolling a die, but also the practice of the expert cannot be judged to be better than that of the novice.

For the practitioner who has doubts about the ability of science to provide all the answers but is concerned about the 'anything goes' attitude of many of its critics, neither of these positions is satisfactory. This, in a nutshell, is the problem that this book attempts to tackle:

how to reject the 'one truth' argument of positivism without falling into the extreme relativism of the 'no truth' argument advocated by some postmodernists. The solution that I offer here is the so-called ironist position, which recognizes the futility of attempting to uncover a single truth, but which nevertheless argues that it is possible to commit oneself to a moral and epistemological stance with integrity and good faith. I attempt to argue, in effect, that although we can never be certain of what is true, we are still able to make choices.

However, in order fully to appreciate postmodern ironism, it is necessary to have some understanding of the philosophical positions that it attempts to undermine. The aim of Part I is therefore to provide a firm grounding in postmodernist philosophy in order to prepare the reader for a detailed and in-depth examination of the postmodern turn in nursing and research in the second part of the book. The first two chapters of Part I examine the two conceptions of truth suggested by the modernist and postmodernist approaches. In Chapter One, the modernist project is described, its history being traced from the time of Bacon and Galileo to the present, including the post-positivist critique. In Chapter Two, the many conflicting notions of postmodernism are explored, and a degree of consensus is achieved concerning the relationship between postmodernism, power and truth. In Chapter Three, the idea of the postmodern ironist is introduced in an attempt to reconcile these two opposing doctrines. Part I ends with a description of the ironist researcher, which provides the foundation for much of what follows in Part II.

NOTES

1. Blake, W. *The Marriage of Heaven and Hell*, 1793.
2. Schön, for example, noted that 'the greater one's proximity to basic science, as a rule, the higher one's academic status', resulting in a 'yearning for the rigor of science-based knowledge and the power of science-based technique'. Schön, D. *Educating the Reflective Practitioner*, San Francisco: Jossey-Bass, 1987.
3. If you feel that this book is already starting to use terminology with which you are unfamiliar, don't worry. All the ideas and concepts that are briefly mentioned in this introduction will be properly introduced and explored in a methodical way in Part I.
4. See, for example, Clarke, L. The last post? Defending nursing against the postmodernist maze, *Journal of Psychiatric and Mental Health Nursing*, 1996, **3**, 257–65; Kermode, S. and Brown, C. The postmodernist hoax and its effect on nursing, *International Journal of Nursing Studies*, 1996, **33**, 4, 375–84.

CHAPTER ONE

Modernism: the rise of empirical research

What is now proved was once only imagin'd[1]

BEFORE MODERNISM

Until the sixteenth century, the concept of truth was largely unproblematic for the majority of people in the West, and was based on a firm and literal belief in Christianity and the Bible. It is tempting to think that the reason for this was simply that people were gullible, that they believed all they were told, particularly where religion was concerned, or else that they were too scared by threats of punishment (in this life and/or the next) *not* to believe. Thus, it was widely accepted as fact that the world was created by God in six days, that we were all descended from Adam and Eve, and that the Earth was the stationary centre of the universe. Even great thinkers such as René Descartes (1596–1650), who is sometimes credited as being the founding father of modern philosophy, based his revolutionary 'method of doubt' on an unshakeable belief in God.[2]

This notion that people were too naïve or too stupid to question the prevailing religious *Zeitgeist* is perhaps itself a rather naïve assumption. Thus, the French philosopher Michel Foucault argued that each age is underpinned by an intellectual 'archive' of knowledge, beliefs and assumptions, an *episteme* that conditions thought to such an extent that it is almost impossible to transcend it. The people of the sixteenth century were therefore no more stupid than the people of today; it is simply that, like us, their thought was restricted to the *episteme* of their time (the Renaissance), which Foucault termed 'resemblance'.[3]

The *episteme* of resemblance was taken by Foucault to mean a resemblance between words and things, such that 'nature and the word can intertwine with one another to infinity, forming, for those who can read it, one vast single text'.[4] The world, then, could be read as a book: as God's book, written in God's language. Thus:

The names of things were lodged in the things they designated, just as strength is written in the body of the lion, regality in the eye of the eagle, just as the influence of the planets is marked upon the brows of men: by the form of similitude.[5]

This simple 'similitude' (similarity of appearance) between what a thing was and the language by which the concept of that thing was expressed, led to a very straightforward notion of truth. Simply by speaking or (more importantly for Foucault) writing, for example, the word 'horse', the very essence of a horse was articulated; it was impossible, when uttering the word 'horse', not to express the truth of the concept of a horse. There was in the sixteenth century, then, 'a non-distinction between what is seen and what is read, between observation and relation, which results in the constitution of a single, unbroken surface in which observation and language intersect to infinity'.[6]

For Foucault, *epistemes* do not gradually shift, but instead follow one another in 'leaps', 'ruptures' or 'mutations'. Thus, at some point in the seventeenth century, the 'resemblance' *episteme* of the Renaissance suddenly gave way to the 'representation' *episteme* of the Classical Age in which 'the profound kinship of language with the world was thus dissolved'.[7] Words no longer resembled things in the world, but merely represented them; there was a schism between the sign and what it signified, so that 'Things and words were to be separated from one another. The eye was thenceforth destined to see and only to see, the ear to hear and only to hear.'[8]

Truth was thus separated from language: in the classical age, the word 'horse' no longer expressed the essence of a horse, but was merely an *abstract* symbol that signified an object in the *concrete* world. If we wished to understand the truth of a horse, we would have to step beyond the abstract world of words and into the concrete world of things. It was only once this episteme of representation became established that empirical science was able to flourish, and with it, the project of modernism.

THE MODERNIST PROJECT

The terms 'modernist', 'modernity' and 'modernism' should not be confused with the more common term 'modern', although they all have their roots in the Latin *modo*, meaning 'just now'. To be modern is to be up to date or in fashion, whereas to be modernist is, ironically, usually considered to be out of date or rooted in the past. The reason for this discrepancy is that the concept to which the word 'modern' refers is constantly changing: what was described as modern twenty years ago is now old fashioned; what is described as modern today will be old fashioned in twenty years time. Indeed, there is evidence to suggest that the term 'modern' (in its Latin form *modernus*) has been in use since at least the fifth century, when it was employed to differentiate between the Christian present and the Roman and pagan past;[9] that is, what to us is fifteen hundred years old was once referred to as being modern.

The concept that the term 'modernist' describes is, however, fixed (although, as we shall see, there is dispute over exactly what it is), referring to a specific historical period rather than an ever-changing now. In the arts, the modernist period usually refers to the first half of the twentieth century, and has been described as 'that earthquake in the arts which brought down much of the structure of pre-twentieth-century practice in music, painting, literature and architecture'.[10] For artists, then, the modernist age is at once a period of innovation and new ideas, as well as a historical period that has now been superseded.

Philosophers, on the other hand, particularly those philosophers known as the postmodernists, usually define modernism in terms of epistemology[11] rather than as an artistic movement. Thus, for the French philosopher Jean-François Lyotard, the term 'modern' is used to designate 'any science that legitimates itself with reference to a metadiscourse... making an explicit appeal to some grand narrative'.[12]

The terms 'metadiscourse' and 'grand narrative' have to be understood in relation to the idea of a discourse and a narrative. A discourse is, loosely speaking, a set of rules or assumptions for organizing and interpreting the subject matter of an academic discipline or field of study.[13] A *meta*discourse, then, goes *beyond* or stands *outside* individual discourses, providing a global rather than a local interpretation of what a discipline should be and how it should organize itself.

Similarly, a narrative is a 'story' that explains the world from a particular perspective, and a *grand* narrative is the story of all the individual narratives, and attempts to fit them together in a coherent whole, an explanation that unites a number of different and possibly contradictory stories or perspectives. Thus, 'By metanarratives or grand narratives, I mean precisely narratives with a legitimizing function.'[14] For Lyotard, then, a modern discourse is one that justifies or legitimates itself with reference to a metadiscourse, that is, to a wider and overarching explanation of how that discourse should generate and validate its knowledge base.

Seen in this way, modernism has been with us since the dawn of recorded history, and is most clearly exemplified in the discourses of religion. For example, the cosmological discourse predominant in sixteenth-century Europe was of the Earth as the centre of the universe, around which all the stars and planets revolved. This discourse was justified not by its internal logic, nor by observations of the external world (both of which were, by this time, beginning to break down), but by an appeal to the metadiscourse of the Christian religion, which emphasized the special and central position of man[15] in creation. A modernist discourse, then, is characterized by its reliance on a higher metadiscourse that is not empirically verifiable and cannot be challenged by logic or reason.

Although, arguably, modernism has always been with us, the period nowadays referred to as modernity is usually thought to begin with the so-called Enlightenment of the eighteenth century.[16] Thus:

> The question of modernity and its consequences is effectively a question of the post-Enlightenment development of Western civilization and the rationalizing project with which it has been articulated. Since the eighteenth century there has been a prominent assumption that increasing rationality is conducive to the promotion of order and control, achievement of enhanced levels of social understanding, moral progress, justice, and human happiness. The pursuit of order, promotion of calculability, fabrication and celebration of the 'new', and faith in 'progress' have been identified as pivotal features of modernity.[17]

This 'Enlightenment narrative'[18] of progress through rationality began as a philosophical movement that included John Locke (1632–1704) and David Hume (1711–1776).[19] It was no less than a 'grand attempt to discover all nature's secrets, including those of humanity',[20] and was characterized by 'a tendency to apply the methods of the new sciences of the age of Newton to other intellectual and philosophical problems'.[21] These Enlightenment philosophers were usually referred to as the empiricists, their position being nicely encapsulated in Hume's invocation that:

> If we take in our hand any volume; of divinity, or school metaphysic, for instance; let us ask, Does it contain any abstract reasoning concerning quantity or number? No. Does it contain any experimental reasoning concerning matters of fact? No. Commit it then to the flames, for it can contain nothing but sophistry and illusion.[22]

For Hume, then, the grand narrative of religion had no solid foundation, and was therefore 'nothing but sophistry and illusion'. We should trust only those things which can be observed and measured, not just in the sciences, but also in philosophy and hence in all aspects of life. Similarly, John Locke saw the human mind as a blank sheet of paper, a *tabula rasa* to be filled by knowledge and ideas 'painted on it with almost endless variety'. As to the question of where this knowledge comes from: 'To this, I answer in one word, from EXPERIENCE; in that all our knowledge is founded, and from that it ultimately derives itself.'[23]

Furthermore, we can see that, for the empiricists, experimental reasoning brought with it a certainty that religion and metaphysics could not guarantee, and was therefore seen as a progression in human thought that contributed to the 'successful forward march of science'.[24] The assumption underpinning the Enlightenment movement, and modernism in general, is one of progress towards some ideal state; that the modern (what we *now* believe) is better than the 'old fashioned' (what we *used* to believe before we knew better).

THE FORWARD MARCH OF SCIENCE

The early inductivists

The Enlightenment project, then, is usually associated with progress through the growth of science and an emphasis on the validation of knowledge through experience, that is, of empirical research. However, the origins of the scientific method stretch back more than a century before the Enlightenment, and are usually attributed to Francis Bacon (1561–1626) and Galileo Galilei (1564–1642), who is particularly remembered for his scientific challenge to the grand narrative of religion. Even before this time, however, Leonardo da Vinci (1452–1519) had set out the basic tenet of empiricism in his claim that 'experience never deceives, it is our judgement only that deceives us, expecting from experience that which is not in its power'.[25] However, it was Galileo and Bacon who developed the systematic approach to collecting those experiences and rationalizing our judgement that has come to be known as the scientific method. Thus, Galileo is credited with founding 'the first school... where all methods other than experiment and calculation were rejected with philosophical severity'.[26]

But if Galileo pioneered the scientific method, then Bacon, who has been referred to as 'the first philosopher of science',[27] outlined the logic that underpinned it. This logic was the logic of induction, which in simple terms is the generalization from a finite number of specific

instances to a general conclusion.[28] Thus, from the fact that the sun
has risen in the east on a number of observed occasions, we might
induce the general law that it always rises in the east. However, Bacon
was not happy with this simple form of 'enumerative' induction:

> For the induction of which the logicians speak, which proceeds by
> simple enumeration, is a puerile thing; concludes at hazard; is always
> liable to be upset by a contradictory instance; takes into account only
> what is known and ordinary; and leads to no result.[29]

Instead, 'what the sciences stand in need of is a form of induction
which shall analyse experience and take it to pieces, and by a due
process of exclusion and rejection lead to an inevitable conclusion'.[30]
Bacon was suggesting that, rather than merely counting up cases,
data should be organized systematically into a number of 'Tables',
including 'Essence and Presence' (a list of cases in which the phenomenon under investigation is present), 'Deviation, or of Absence in
Proximity' (cases in which the phenomenon is absent) and 'Degrees,
or Comparisons' (cases in which the phenomenon is present to
varying degrees).[31]

Having assembled these tables, it would then be possible to compare
cases between them and arrive at some logical conclusions about the
phenomenon under investigation. For example, if we wished to explore
the phenomenon of magnetism, we might draw up a Table of Presence
of all the materials that are magnetic, and a Table of Absence of all the
materials that are not magnetic. From these, we might notice that all
the materials in the Table of Presence contained iron, whereas none of
the materials in the Table of Absence did so. Thus, we might conclude
that the presence of iron is associated with magnetism, and further test
this theory by examining the Table of Comparisons to see whether
materials that contain large amounts of iron are more magnetic than
those which contain small amounts of iron.

Bacon thought that he had discovered a scientific method that, if
properly applied, would guarantee accurate findings. The senses, he
claimed, were easily deceived, so:

> To meet these difficulties, I have sought on all sides diligently and faith-
> fully to provide helps for the sense – substitutes to supply its failures,
> rectifications to correct its errors; and this I endeavour to accomplish
> not so much by instruments as by experiments.[32]

Bacon's method was widely adopted by seventeenth-century
scientists, including Robert Hooke (1635–1703), Robert Boyle
(1627–1691) and Isaac Newton (1642–1727). Newton in particular

followed Bacon's experimental approach of rejecting non-empirical hypotheses in favour of a purely inductive methodology such that:

> hypotheses, whether metaphysical or physical, whether of occult quali-
> ties or mechanical, have no place in experimental philosophy. In this
> philosophy particular propositions are inferred from the phenomena,
> and afterwards rendered general by induction.[33]

The origins of social science

A later advocate of Bacon's method was Auguste Comte (1798–1857), who is widely acknowledged as the founder of modern social science, and who coined the terms 'positivism' and 'sociology'. His programme of 'extending Bacon's conception of the study of nature to the social'[34] was later taken up by, among others, the philosopher John Stuart Mill (1806–1873) and the sociologist Emile Durkheim (1858–1917), who both wanted to build a social science on the same solid foundations as those of the natural sciences.[35]

Mill, probably more than Comte, took Bacon's inductive science to its logical conclusion. He postulated a number of 'methods' similar to Bacon's three Tables, which he called the 'method of agreement', the 'method of differences', the 'joint method of agreement and difference' and the 'method of concomitant variations'.[36] Furthermore, like Newton, Mill considered hypothesizing to have no place in the scientific method, particularly in the social sciences, favouring what he called 'pure induction', which he defined as:

> the process by which we conclude that what is true of certain individ-
> uals of a class is true of the whole class, or that what is true at certain
> times will be true in similar circumstances at all times.[37]

Mill's attempt to apply Bacon's inductive methods of the pure sciences to sociology[38] has been described as a 'bottom-up' approach[39] because it argues that general laws about the workings of society are derived from 'the laws of individual human nature',[40] such that 'Human beings in society have no properties but those which are derived from, and may be resolved into, the laws of nature of individual man.'[41] Mill has sometimes been accused of sociological psychologism – the view that sociological explanations can be reduced to individual mental phenomena – and it is probably true that Mill's account of social events owes more to psychology than it does to sociology.

Mill's view is contrasted with the 'top-down' approach advocated by social scientists such as L.-A.-J. Quetelet (1796–1874), who argued that by studying the characteristics of large numbers of individuals, it was possible to build theories inductively about the 'average man', and while individual differences might assert some influence in specific cases:

> every thing which pertains to the human species considered as a whole, belongs to the order of physical facts: the greater the number of individuals, the more does the influence of individual will disappear, leaving predominance to a series of general facts, dependant on causes by which society exists and is preserved.[42]

Others went even further. Henry Thomas Buckle (1821–1862), for example, wrote in 1861 that the statistical approach to the study of society led to the conclusion that:

> the actions of men, being determined solely by their antecedents, must have a character of uniformity, that is to say, must, under precisely the same circumstances, always issue in precisely the same results'.[43]

This top-down approach to the study of society met with some early success, and led to a number of theories and predictions about the behaviour of large groups of people, for example Durkheim's attempt to correlate suicide rates with different national, religious and social variables.[44] However, Durkheim himself was very aware of the limits of this new discipline of sociology. It could not, for example, provide any information about the suicidal behaviour of individuals – that was the task of biology or medicine – so Quetelet's project to develop a measure of the probability of any particular individual committing suicide was dismissed by Durkheim as not being true sociology. For Durkheim, the whole was more than the sum of its parts, and 'society is not a mere sum of individuals... the system formed by their association represents a specific reality which has its own characteristics'.[45]

Even Mill, who was advocating a bottom-up approach in which the micro level of the individual determined behaviour at the macro level of society, recognized the theoretical poverty of a simple enumerative model of induction. Thus, he pointed out that:

> What is obtained, even after the most extensive and accurate observation, is merely a comparative result; as, for example, that in a given number of Frenchmen, taken indiscriminately, there will be found more persons of a particular mental tendency, and fewer of the contrary tendency, than among an equal number of Italians or English, similarly taken.[46]

The seemingly facile outcome of this statistical approach to the study of society was later addressed in a more constructive fashion by Max Weber (1864–1920), another influential early sociologist. For Weber, the focus of sociology was not Quetelet's 'average man', a distillation of a large number of statistical data, but rather the 'ideal type'.[47] The difference between the average man and the ideal type is subtle but important, both, for example, representing abstractions rather than actual living people, but whereas Quetelet's average man was a *statistical* generalization from the behaviour of a large number of individuals, Weber's ideal type was an *analytic* generalization[48] to a theoretical construct. Ideal types, then, 'are concepts intended to make it possible to bring order to the chaos of individual historical facts'.[49]

Furthermore, the study of ideal types has a moral component: it is concerned less with describing how the world is than with how it ought to be, asking the question 'How should we live?'[50] But if the aim of sociology is to explore theoretical and moral concepts rather than to construct statistical composites, the overtly scientific macro methods advocated by Durkheim will not do. Thus, in response to the question of how we should live, Weber acknowledged that 'The fact that science does not give us this answer is completely undeniable.'[51]

In fact, Weber questioned the whole enterprise of nineteenth-century positivist sociology. Since sociology grew out of the physical sciences, it retained the broad aim of the explanation (*Erklären*) of social behaviour. However, Weber believed that the social sciences should aim not merely to explain, but to understand (*Verstehen*),[52] to 'accomplish something which is never attainable in the natural sciences, namely the subjective understanding of the action of the component individuals'.[53] This understanding of individuals can clearly never be attained through the study of large groups, but requires an individual approach, and the challenge of this 'science of the singular'[54] has been taken up through the development of research methods such as phenomenology, ethnography, action research and case study. Weber's distinction between *Erklären* and *Verstehen* therefore triggered a schism in sociology that has still not been resolved, and has almost resulted in two sociologies: an objective, quantitative paradigm and a more subjective, qualitative one.

The pragmatists

By the mid-nineteenth century, however, the physical sciences were moving away from pure inductivism towards a composite method that involved both inductive and deductive logic. The reason for this can be seen partly in the shift in the prevailing philosophical mood from idealism to utilitarianism.[55] Thus, the driving force behind the development of science moved away from metaphysical speculation on the nature of knowledge and reality towards the political concept of the greatest happiness of the greatest number. Science was no longer the province of the idle rich, who inductively collected 'facts' in the same way that they collected jewellery or fine clothes, but became linked to technology and utility. Scientists no longer had the luxury of fitting together the findings from disjointed experiments like pieces of a jigsaw, in the hope that they might form a coherent picture. What the ever-growing industrial revolution demanded was not just a method of science, but a method of scientific discovery, a method of optimizing the chances of uncovering *useful* findings.

This new method rejected the *ad hoc* collection of empirical data in favour of the purposeful collection of data in order to prove a specific hypothesis. The philosopher Charles Peirce (1839–1914) argued that this method involved three logical processes: first, *abduction*, or inference to the best explanation: the postulation of a hypothesis to explain a particular phenomenon; second, *deduction* of the consequences that might follow if the hypothesis were correct; and third, *induction* to test those consequences through the collection of empirical data.[56] Peirce was the originator of the philosophical doctrine of pragmatism, which argued that the truth of a concept should be defined by the practical consequences of its application rather than by some intrinsic property that it possesses. Thus, for William James (1842–1910), another pragmatist, '"the true", to put it very briefly, is only the expedient in the way of our thinking, just as "the right" is only the expedient in the way of our behaving'.[57] Science was therefore less to do with truth and certainty than with what worked in the real world.

The contrast between these two approaches to science, eighteenth-century idealism and nineteenth-century pragmatism, can be seen in their respective attitudes towards the so-called 'problem of induction'. Hume, who we have already seen was one of the original Enlightenment philosophers and a strict empiricist, was well aware that inductive reasoning could not be relied upon to produce accurate findings.[58] Through a rather complex argument, he demonstrated that inductive inferences are not logically justified, but that they rely on custom or habit. We therefore have no firm grounds for inferring the future from the past, or that cases we have not observed will resemble cases we have observed.

This, of course, presented an enormous problem for Hume, who, you might recall, wanted to consign to the flames any book that did not contain abstract or experimental reasoning. Thus, as the philosopher Karl Popper (1902–1994) pointed out:

> By these results Hume himself – one of the most rational minds ever – was turned into a sceptic and, at the same time, into a believer: a believer in an irrationalist epistemology. His result that repetition has no power whatever in an argument, although it dominates our cognitive life or our 'understanding', led him to the conclusion that argument or reason plays only a minor role in our understanding. Our 'knowledge' is unmasked as being not only of the nature of belief, but of rationally indefensible belief – of *an irrational faith*.[59]

Hume, then, lost his faith in science not because it failed to work, but because it was philosophically and logically flawed.

In contrast, the logical uncertainties introduced by the problem of induction mattered little to the pragmatists, since 'fallible and imperfect as scientific inquiry is, however, if this vast co-operative enterprise were to continue long enough... eventually a final, stable opinion would be reached'.[60] Inductive science might occasionally fail, but in the long run it will serve its pragmatic purpose of technological advancement: if it works in practice, there is no need to fix it.[61]

Hypothetico-deductivism and the logical positivists

We have already seen that Popper was rather scathing of Hume's inductivism, and his colleague Bertrand Russell (1872–1970) was equally dismissive, stating that 'Hume's philosophy... represents the bankruptcy of eighteenth-century reasonableness',[62] and adding that if Hume were right, 'every attempt to arrive at general scientific laws from particular observations is fallacious, and Hume's scepticism is inescapable for an empiricist'.[63]

The inevitable conclusion of Hume's problem of induction was that the whole of Western science is built on unsound reasoning, and in particular, that the so-called truths arrived at by the scientific method were in fact not truths at all. As Popper went on to point out, 'we must regard all laws or theories as hypothetical or conjectural; that is, as guesses',[64] and the fact that the sun has risen in the east every morning since the dawn of recorded history is no guarantee that it will rise in the east tomorrow.

Nor was Peirce's pragmatism any more reassuring, since taken to its logical conclusion, 'almost any belief might be respectable, and even true, provided it works'.[65] Both the idealist and the pragmatist accounts of induction therefore lead inevitably to a subjectivism that, for a number of twentieth-century philosophers including Popper and the logical positivists,[66] was totally unacceptable.

Popper attempted to resolve the issue not by denying or refuting the problem of induction, but by claiming that science does not, after all, depend on inductive logic. Instead, he claimed, it proceeds according to the method of falsification or what has come to be known as hypothetico-deductivism. The hypothetico-deductive method has been described as '(1) setting up a hypothesis, (2) deducing consequences from the hypothesis, and (3) checking by observation to see whether these consequences are true'.[67] For example, I might advance the hypothesis that all swans are white, and deduce that, if this were indeed the case, every observed swan anywhere in the world would be white. Thus, every report that came in of a white swan would lend support to my hypothesis, while competing hypotheses such as that all swans have orange beaks would fall by the wayside. Finally, however, a report of a black swan might be received, in which case my hypothesis would have to be rejected, or at least modified to take account of white *and* black swans.

Popper's hypothetico-deductivism might appear similar to Peirce's 'abduction–deduction–induction' model described earlier. However, Popper claimed that it is different in two respects. First, the initial stage of abducing a hypothesis is omitted; for Popper, hypotheses appear fully formed to the scientist. Second, Peirce's inductive stage, in which evidence is collected to prove a hypothesis (and in which the problem of induction is introduced into the process) is replaced by a falsification stage.

Thus, Popper argued that although no amount of confirmatory cases can ever *prove* a hypothesis, it takes only one disconfirmatory case to *disprove* it. How ever many white swans I observe, there is always the chance that the next one I see will be black, or red, or purple. Therefore, although I can never prove the hypothesis that all swans are white, and hence it can never become a scientific law, I only need to observe one purple swan to *disprove* the hypothesis.[68]

For Popper, then, the aim of science is not to attempt to prove a hypothesis, but to attempt to disprove it, and the demarcation between what is a scientific hypothesis and what is not, is that a scientific hypothesis is capable of being disproved by deducing consequences of the hypothesis for testing. Thus, competing hypotheses are weeded out, and those which survive all attempts to disprove them can be tentatively accepted as closer to the truth than those which do not survive. Scientific knowledge therefore evolves in a Darwinian way as a survival-of-the-fittest hypothesis.

Popper thought that, by replacing inductivism with hypothetico-deductivism, he had solved a great philosophical problem and put science back on a sound empirical foundation. For the inductivists, nothing is certain, and any scientific theory is liable to topple at any time. Through the method of hypothetico-deductivism, Popper believed that he had introduced a systematic way of weeding out the weaker theories, so that although we can never be absolutely certain that we have discovered the truth, we can nevertheless have good grounds for suspecting that we have. Thus:

> We test for truth, by eliminating falsehood. That we cannot give a justification – or sufficient reasons – for our guesses does not mean that we may not have guessed the truth; some of our hypotheses may well be true.[69]

However, Popper's solution to the problem of induction has been criticized on both logical and practical grounds. In terms of logic, Popper argued that we should regard highly corroborated theories (that is, theories that have survived many tests of falsification) as more likely to be true than theories that are not so highly corroborated. But as Gower pointed out, when we say of a theory that it is highly corroborated, 'we are reporting on its past success in passing severe tests, which cannot be a good ground for Popper to declare that it will in future pass other severe tests'.[70] Clearly, then, Popper's alternative to inductivism is itself based partly on inductive logic, and the fact that a theory has survived a large number of tests of falsification in the past provides us with no grounds for thinking that it will continue to survive such tests in the future.

In addition, on practical grounds, Kuhn, Feyerabend and others have pointed out that Popper might well have formulated *a* logic of scientific discovery, but it was not *the* logic employed by most practising scientists. Thus, 'No process yet disclosed by the historical study of scientific development at all resembles the methodological stereotypes of falsification by direct comparison with nature.'[71] Rather ironically, then, while Popper's methods of falsification and hypothetico-deductivism have been heavily criticized, his cautious scepticism has been misinterpreted by some writers as an out-and-out denial of scientific truth.[72]

TOWARDS A POST-POSITIVISM

From as early as the 1950s, empiricism in general, and positivism in particular, was being attacked from within. Willard van Orman Quine (1908–), for example, was originally a student of the logical positivist Rudolf Carnap (1891–1970), but later produced a radical critique of his early position. In the paper 'Two dogmas of empiricism', Quine argued against the notion of empirical observations of a 'real' world as objective verification of scientific theories. Instead, all observation is itself theory-laden, and empirical science is therefore an holistic web of beliefs, 'a man made fabric which impinges on experience only along the edges'.[73] However, by the 1960s, the focus for post-positivist philosophers of science such as Thomas Kuhn (1922–) had switched from the nature of science to the nature of truth. Earlier writers such as Popper accepted that objective independent truth existed (he even created a 'world' for it);[74] what was in dispute was the scientific methods for gaining access to that truth. However, for Kuhn, the 'truth' was dependant on the rules and methods (loosely referred to as paradigms) employed in seeking it out. Thus:

> one of the things a scientific community acquires with a paradigm is a criterion for choosing problems that, while the paradigm is taken for granted, can be assumed to have solutions. To a great extent these are the only problems that the community will admit as scientific or encourage its members to undertake. Other problems... are rejected as metaphysical, as the concern of another discipline, or sometimes as just too problematic to be worth the time.[75]

The scientific community, through its choice of paradigm, defines the scope of what it considers to be 'real' science, and thereby defines the scope of what counts as scientific truth. Most of the time spent by most scientists is devoted to reinforcing the dominant paradigm by 'puzzle solving',[76] in which puzzles are problems that are defined by the rules of the paradigm and are assured of solutions. Thus, much of the effort of scientists is expended in the 'mopping up operations' of filling in the missing parts of the puzzle, what Kuhn referred to as 'normal science'.[77]

However, from time to time, the established paradigm undergoes a radical shift brought about by the failure of the solutions to puzzles to come out in the ways predicted by that paradigm. Scientists usually cling on to the established paradigm for as long as they can, often in the face of growing evidence that it no longer adequately explains or predicts the world. Eventually, however, the evidence against it becomes so strong that it breaks down, and a new paradigm is established. Kuhn referred to these sudden shifts as 'scientific revolutions'. The implication, then, is that there is no objective scientific truth, but that the truth shifts along with the paradigms employed for uncovering it. As the physicist Werner Heisenberg pointed out, 'What we observe is not nature itself, but nature exposed to our method of questioning.'[78]

For Kuhn, however, it was not simply a matter of an inadequate paradigm being replaced by a better one, but rather that 'the competition between paradigms is not the sort of battle that can be resolved by proofs',[79] and therefore 'we may... have to relinquish the notion, explicit or implicit, that changes of paradigm carry scientists closer to the truth'[80] Implicit in Kuhn's view of science, then, is a critique of the possibility of scientific progress and hence of the Enlightenment project itself.

Paul Feyerabend (1924–1994) developed Kuhn's notion of scientific paradigms further to consider the ways in which they constrain scientists in their everyday work. For Kuhn, a paradigm includes 'law, theory, application, and instrumentation together';[81] that is, it determines not only the kind of puzzles that are considered appropriate for the scientist to work on, but also the methods by which those puzzles should be tackled. This has advantages, since:

> By placing a heavy emphasis on correct method, all members of a scientific community are assured a kind of collective protection: madmen, charlatans, fakers, and sophists are hopefully excluded from the ranks.[82]

But there is a twofold price to be paid for this security. First, as well as excluding madmen and charlatans, this emphasis on method can also be employed to exclude deviants and troublemakers who might have a genuine and valuable contribution to make to the discipline. Second, an overemphasis on correct method can serve to stifle creativity. As Hollis pointed out:

> Young scientists serve apprenticeships, in which they learn to think and practise as required by the prevailing paradigm, and they are promoted for learning the lesson well. The heroic saga of the isolated individual genius is purely a myth.[83]

However, as Feyerabend noted, this system of rules is not intended to describe what scientists *actually* do, but is instead 'supposed to provide us with normative rules which *should* be followed, and to which *actual scientific practice will correspond only more or less closely*'.[84] Furthermore, 'there is not a single rule, however plausible, and however firmly grounded in epistemology, that is not violated at some time or other',[85] and many significant scientific developments 'occurred either because some thinkers decided not to be bound by certain "obvious" methodological rules or because they unwittingly broke them'.[86]

Feyerabend supported this assertion with a number of historical case studies of famous scientists, including Galileo, whom he claimed flaunted every methodological rule in the book and yet is still held up as an exemplar of good science. Similarly, Mitroff examined the ways in which contemporary scientists actually worked, and found that the scientists who were most highly regarded by their colleagues were those who rejected the norms and rigours of scientific method. In contrast, scientists who kept to the rules and adhered to the norms were often dismissed as mere technicians.[87]

Feyerabend therefore advocated a 'methodological anarchism' in which 'There is only *one* principle that can be defended under *all* circumstances and in *all* stages of human development. It is the principle: *anything goes*'.[88] In a similar vein, Albert Einstein observed that:

> The external conditions which are set for [the scientist] by the facts of experience do not permit him to let himself be too much restricted in the construction of his conceptual world by the adherence to an epistemological system. He therefore must appear to the systematic epistemologist as a type of unscrupulous opportunist.[89]

In advocating for methodological anarchism, however, Feyerabend was not seeking to establish a new methodology, yet another of Einstein's epistemological systems; instead, he was expressing 'the terrified exclamation of a rationalist who takes a closer look at history'.[90] He was thus supporting Kuhn's assertion that there is no single set of methodological rules that comprises 'good science', and therefore that no one paradigm is 'better' than any other.

The sociologist C. Wright Mills echoed these sentiments in the social sciences with his notions of the 'sociological imagination' and 'intellectual craftsmanship'.[91] Thus, 'the classic social analyst has avoided any rigid set of procedures; he has sought to develop and use in his work the sociological imagination',[92] and furthermore 'he has not been inhibited by method and technique; the classic way has been the way of the intellectual craftsman'.[93] For Mills, then, the successful social scientist is not bound by any particular method or critique, but devises her own in response to the problem she is tackling. In this, Mills pre-empted Feyerabend's call for methodological anarchism by advocating that:

The slogans we ought to raise are surely these:
Every man his own methodologist!
Methodologists! Get to work![94]

Derek Phillips[95] continued very much from where C. Wright Mills left off, effectively applying the post-positivist arguments of Kuhn and Feyerabend to his own critique of the social sciences. In particular, he attacked the supposed objectivity of the social scientist and her claim that she has available infallible criteria for distinguishing truth from falsity. Phillips drew on the work of the philosopher Ludwig Wittgenstein and his notion of language games, which argues that there are no standards existing outside language that can be used to justify the truth or falsity of a statement. Thus, since language is a human invention, so too is scientific or sociological truth.[96] Put crudely, 'language is more than a means of communicating about reality: it is a tool for constructing reality'.[97] Sociology, therefore, cannot be other than a series of subjective positions, and:

> Although sociologists proceed as if we had access to a neutral, extra-linguistic means of reporting, of talking about truth and knowledge, it seems preferable to recognize that there is no knowledge that is objective or impersonal or guaranteed by a divine mind. Sociological truth and knowledge are human phenomena and are to be found in the cultural milieu, in the tradition, in the form of life of sociology itself.[98]

Even in physics, that most positivist of the hard sciences, subjectivity has began to creep in during the course of the twentieth century, and as Wittgenstein noted:

> The fact that it can be described by Newtonian Mechanics tells us nothing about the world; but this tells us something, namely, that the world can be described in that particular way in which as a matter of fact it is described.[99]

But the fact is, of course, that the world could also be described in numerous other ways. Thus, the physicist Werner Heisenberg pointed out that 'Natural science does not simply describe and explain nature; it is part of the interplay between nature and ourselves',[100] while John Wheeler claimed that:

> Nothing is more important about the quantum principle than this, that it destroys the concept of the world as 'sitting out there', with the observer safely separated from it by a 20 centimeter slab of plate glass. Even to observe so minuscule an object as an electron, he must shatter

the glass. He must reach in. He must install his chosen measuring equipment... Moreover, the measurement changes the state of the electron. The universe will never afterwards be the same.[101]

The above quotation would have horrified David Hume, and would undoubtedly have been committed to the flames as containing 'nothing but sophistry and illusion'. Thus, by the mid-1970s, the modernist project of the Enlightenment, with its mission of boundless and inevitable progress through the certainties of science, had become seriously compromised, to be replaced by a softer, less certain, post-positivist science.

NOTES

1. Blake, W. *The Marriage of Heaven and Hell*, 1793.
2. Descartes begins his philosophical quest by doubting everything, including God. However, as many commentators have pointed out, this is merely a rhetorical device, and 'it is important to realize that Descartes is in no sense a sceptic. The systematic doubt is merely a means to an end: the aim is to demolish in order to rebuild.' Dancy, J. and Sosa, E. *A Companion to Epistemology*, Oxford: Blackwell, 1992, p. 95. Read in this way, the famous *cogito ergo sum* (I think, therefore I exist) is simply the first step in Descartes' real agenda, which was a philosophical proof of the existence of God.
3. Foucault, M. (1966) *The Order of Things: An Archaeology of the Human Sciences*, London: Tavistock, 1974.
4. *Ibid.*, p. 34.
5. *Ibid.*, p. 36.
6. *Ibid.*, p. 39.
7. *Ibid.*, p. 43.
8. *Ibid.*, p. 43.
9. Habermas, J. Modernity – an incomplete project, *New German Critique*, 1981, **22**, 3–15.
10. Barry, P. *Beginning Theory*, Manchester: Manchester University Press, 1995, p. 81.
11. Epistemology can be defined as the study of the way in which knowledge is conceptualized and generated.
12. Lyotard, J.-F. (1979) *The Postmodern Condition: A Report on Knowledge*, Manchester: Manchester University Press, 1984, p. xxiii.
13. Jenkins, K. *Re-thinking History*, London: Routledge, 1991, p. 71. Foucault went further by arguing that discourses do not merely *describe* reality, but 'systematically *form* the objects of which they speak': Foucault, M. (1969) *The Archaeology of Knowledge*, London: Tavistock, 1974, p. 49, emphasis added.

14 Lyotard, J.-F. (1984) Apostil on narratives. In J.-F. Lyotard *The Postmodern Explained to Children*, London: Turnaround, 1992, p. 31.

15. In general, I will use the female gender throughout in an attempt to redress the balance of writings from a male perspective. However, on this occasion, the Christian religion was referring specifically to men rather than to people in general.

16. This period roughly corresponds to Foucault's Classical Age.

17. Smart, B. *Postmodernity*, London: Routledge, 1993, p. 91.

18. Lyotard (1979) *op. cit.*, p. xxiii.

19. Walter Truett Anderson has argued that the Enlightenment project was triggered in the mid-eighteenth century by the young French philosopher A.-R.-J. Turgot (1727–1781), who declared at a public lecture at the Sorbonne that '[humankind] advances ever, though slowly, towards greater perfection'. Anderton, W.T. *The Fontana Postmodernism Reader*, London: Fontana Press, 1996, p. 219.

20. Hollis, M. *The Philosophy of Social Science*, Cambridge: Cambridge University Press, 1994, p. 5.

21. Hamlyn, D.W. *A History of Western Philosophy*, Harmondsworth: Penguin, 1987, p. 206.

22. Hume, D. (1748) *Enquiry Concerning Human Understanding*, Section XII, Part III, London: Longman, 1875.

23. Locke, J. (1690) *Essay Concerning Human Understanding*, Book II, Chapter 1, Section 2, London: Dent, 1961, p. 77; his capitals.

24. Sorell, T. *Scientism: Philosophy and the Infatuation with Science*, London: Routledge, 1991, p. 7.

25. da Vinci, L. (*c.* 1490) *Codex Atlanticus*, unpublished manuscript.

26. Condorcet, Marquis de (1795) *Sketch for a Historical Picture of the Progress of the Human Mind*, S. Hampshire (ed.), J. Barraclough (trans.), London: Weidenfeld & Nicolson, 1955, p. 115.

27. Cranston, M. *Philosophers and Pamphleteers*, Oxford: Oxford University Press, 1985, p. 48.

28. The term 'induction' is used in a number of different ways. Scientific induction is usually characterized by the generation of a theory from data previously collected without a specific hypothesis in mind. Thus, the theory 'emerges' from the data.

29. Bacon, F. (1620) *The Great Instauration*, J. Weinberger (ed.), J. Spedding (trans.), Illinois: Harlan Davidson, 1989, p. 23.

30. *Ibid.*, p. 23.

31. Bacon, F. (1620) *The New Organon and Related Writings*, F.H. Anderson (ed.), New York: Macmillan, 1985.

32. Bacon, F. (1620) *op. cit.*, 1989, p. 24.

33. Newton, I. (1726) *Principia*, Volume 2 (facsimile reprint), A. Motte (trans.), London: Dawsons of Pall Mall, 1968, p. 314.

34. Hughes, J. *The Philosophy of Social Research*, London: Longman, 1990, p. 18.

35. The computer scientist Marvin Minsky, paraphrasing Freud, referred to this tendency as 'physics envy'.

36. Mill, J.S. (1843) *A System of Logic*, 8th edn, London: Longman, 1967, pp. 253–66.

37. *Ibid*, p. 200.

38. The fact that Mill was able to formulate a social science at all is, according to Foucault, the result of a shift in the prevailing *episteme* from the classical to the modern at the start of the nineteenth century. Thus, whereas the classical age is characterized by 'representation' (see the beginning of the chapter), the modern age is the age of 'self-reference' in which there is a total break between words and things. This epistemological break has far-reaching implications; the break between words and what they represent has 'cut free' our language in such a way that words function as 'a self-referential discourse of a transcendental human subject with itself': Kearney, R. *Modern Movements in European Philosophy*, 2nd edn, Manchester: Manchester University Press, 1994, p. 288. For Foucault, the dawn of the modern age heralded the possibility of a concept of man (Foucault's term) as 'an empirical entity' (Foucault, *op. cit.*, p. 344) and therefore as an object of study. Thus, it is only within the modern *episteme* of self-reference that the human sciences such as sociology and psychology have been able to emerge.

39. Hollis, *op. cit.*, p. 16.

40. Mill, *op. cit.*, p. 573.

41. *Ibid*, p. 573.

42. Quetelet, A. (1835) *A Treatise on Man and the Development of his Faculties*, New York: Burt Franklin, 1968, p. 96.

43. Buckle, H.T. *History of Civilization in England*, Volume 1, London: Longmans, 1861, p. 20.

44. Durkheim, E. (1897) *Suicide: A Study in Sociology*, London: Routledge & Kegan Paul, 1952.

45. Durkheim, E. (1895) *The Rules of Sociological Method*, G. Catlin (ed.), New York: Free Press, 1966, pp. 103–4.

46. Mill, *op cit.*, p. 565.

47. Weber, M. (1905) *The Protestant Ethic and the Spirit of Capitalism*, London: Unwin, 1930.

48. An analytic generalization extrapolates from one or more single cases to a theory 'analogous to the way a scientist generalizes from experimental results to a theory': Yin, R.K. *Case Study Research*, London: Sage, 1994, p. 37.

49. Smith, R. *The Fontana History of the Human Sciences*, London: Fontana, 1997, p. 558.

50. Weber, M. (1919) Science as vocation. In P. Lassman and I. Velody, *Max Weber's 'Science as Vocation'*, London: Unwin Hyman, 1989, p. 18.

51. *Ibid*.

52. The terms *Erklären* and *Verstehen* were first employed by the German philosopher and social scientist Wilhelm Dilthey.

53. Weber, M. (1921) *Economy and Society*, Volume 1, New York: Bedminster Press, 1968, p. 15.
54. Simons, H. *Towards a Science of the Singular*, Norwich: University of East Anglia, 1980.
55. Fowler, W.S. *The Development of Scientific Method*, Oxford: Pergamon Press, 1962, p. 66.
56. Peirce, C.S. How to make our ideas clear, *Popular Science Monthly*, 1878, **12**, 286–302.
57. James, W. *Pragmatism*, London: Longman, 1907, p. 222. James in fact went further by linking the concept of truth not only with expediency, but also with moral good. Thus, 'In the case of truth, untrue beliefs work as perniciously in the long run as true beliefs work beneficially... the one may be called good, the other bad, unconditionally.' *Ibid.*, p. 231.
58. Hume, *op. cit.*
59. Popper, K.R. (1972) *Objective Knowledge*, rev. edn, Oxford: Clarendon Press, 1979, pp. 4–5, original emphasis.
60. Haack, S. Entry on Peirce. In J. Dancy and E. Sosa (eds) *A Companion to Epistemology*, Oxford: Blackwell, 1993, p. 353.
61. The effectiveness of this pragmatic approach to science is clearly evident in the explosion of scientific discovery during the nineteenth century, culminating in the industrialization of the Western world.
62. Russell, B. *A History of Western Philosophy*, London: Allen & Unwin, 1946, p. 698.
63. *Ibid.*, p. 698.
64. Popper, *op. cit.*, p. 9. Popper first expressed this view in Popper, K.R. (1935) *The Logic of Scientific Discovery*, London: Hutchinson, 1959.
65. Blackburn, S. *The Oxford Dictionary of Philosophy*, Oxford: OUP, 1994, p. 297.
66. Logical positivism, which included the early philosophy of Wittgenstein along with that of Russell and Ayer, combined linguistic logic with a strong scientific empiricism.
67. Salmon, W. *Logic*, Englewood Cliffs: Prentice Hall, 1963, p. 78.
68. Although Popper presented the method of falsification as a breakthrough in the philosophy of science, it had been known of for at least three hundred years. Thus, Galileo wrote that: 'I know very well that one single experiment or conclusive proof to the contrary would be enough to batter to the ground... a great many probable arguments': Galileo (1629) *Dialogue Concerning Two Chief World Systems*, 2nd rev. edn, S. Drake (trans.), California: University of California Press, 1967. Popper's real breakthrough was in claiming that falsification avoided the need for induction.
69. Popper, *op. cit.*, 1972, p. 30.
70. Gower, B. *Scientific Method*, London: Routledge, 1997, p. 207.
71. Kuhn, T.S. *The Structure of Scientific Revolutions*, Chicago: University of Chicago Press, 1962, p. 77.

72. As Popper himself rather peevishly pointed out in a footnote in one of his books (Popper, *op. cit.*, 1972), 'the *Encyclopedia of Philosophy*... attributes to me the view: "Truth itself is just an illusion"'.

73. Quine, W.V.O. (1953) Two dogmas of empiricism. In W.V.O. Quine, *From a Logical Point of View*, Cambridge MA: Harvard University Press, 1980, p. 42.

74. Popper postulated three 'worlds'. World 1 was the world of physical objects, World 2 was the mental world of subjective thought, belief and experience, and World 3 was the world of objective thought and knowledge.

75. Kuhn, *op. cit.*, p. 37.

76. *Ibid.*, p. 36.

77. *Ibid.*, p. 38.

78. Heisenberg, W. *Physics and Philosophy*, London: Allen & Unwin, 1963, p. 57.

79. Kuhn, *op. cit.*, p. 147.

80. *Ibid.*, p. 119. Kuhn suggested that paradigms are incommensurate with one another, that meaningful dialogue between paradigms, and hence agreement on what counts as truth, is impossible.

81. *Ibid.*, p. 10.

82. Phillips, D.L. *Abandoning Method*, London: Jossey-Bass, 1973, p. 154.

83. Hollis, M. *The Philosophy of Social Science*, Cambridge: Cambridge University Press, 1994, p. 86.

84. Feyerabend, P.K. Explanation, reduction, and empiricism. In H. Feigl and G. Maxwell (eds) *Scientific Explanation, Space, and Time: Minnesota Studies in the Philosophy of Science*, Volume 3, Minneapolis: University of Minnesota Press, 1962, p. 60, emphasis added.

85. Feyerabend, P.K. *Against Method*, London: Verso, 1975, p. 23.

86. *Ibid.*, p. 24.

87. Mitroff, I. *The Scientific Side of Science*, Amsterdam: Elsevier, 1974.

88. Feyerabend, *op. cit.*, pp. 18–19, original emphasis.

89. Cited in Schlipp, P.A. *Albert Einstein, Philosopher-Scientist*, Evanston, IL: Tudor, 1948, p. 683.

90. Feyerabend, P.K. *Against Method*, 3rd edn, London: Verso, 1993, p. vii.

91. Mills, C.W. (1959) *The Sociological Imagination*, Harmondsworth: Penguin, 1970.

92. *Ibid.*, p. 134.

93. *Ibid.*, p. 134.

94. *Ibid.*, p. 137.

95. Phillips, *op. cit.*

96. This is a grossly oversimplified summary of Wittgenstein's position, which will be explored more fully in Chapter Three. A scholarly analysis of the role of language games in the social sciences can also be found in Winch, P. *The Idea of a Social Science and its Relation to Philosophy*, 2nd edn, London: Routledge, 1990.

97. Spradley, J. *The Ethnographic Interview*, New York: Holt, Rinehart & Winston, 1979, p. 17.
98. Phillips, *op. cit.*, p. 150.
99. Wittgenstein, L. *Tractatus Logico-Philosophicus*, London: Kegan Paul, 1922, p. 342.
100. Heisenberg, *op. cit.*, p. 75.
101. In J. Mehra (ed.) *The Physicist's Conception of Nature*, Dordrecht, Holland: Reidel, 1973, p. 244.

CHAPTER TWO

Postmodernism: the challenge to empirical research

Without contraries is no progression[1]

THE POSTMODERNIST CRITIQUE

In the previous chapter, I explored a number of critiques of the modernist position, and in particular, of empirical science, the principal method for driving modernism forward. However, all of these critiques originated from within the modernist movement itself, and the target of their criticism was not empirical research *per se*, but the way in which that research is usually thought to be conducted. Thus, as the titles of their books suggest, Feyerabend was *against method*, rather than against science, and Phillips advocated *abandoning method*, rather than abandoning science. Similarly, Kuhn's *scientific revolutions* were revolutions *within* the scientific community rather than revolutions against science, and his postulated paradigm shifts all took place safely inside the metaparadigm of science. In fact, in his later work, Kuhn to some extent recanted his earlier relativist position.[2]

All of the above writers were essentially modernists, albeit post-positivist modernists, in as much as they subscribed to the Enlightenment project of inexorable progress towards the universal good. What these writers were challenging was not so much the ends of science as the means by which those ends could most effectively be achieved.

A more serious critique comes from outside the metaparadigm of science, and is a critique not merely of the scientific method, but of the ends of science, and indeed, of modernism itself. This critique of 'the Enlightenment narrative, in which the hero of knowledge works towards a good ethico-political end – universal peace'[3] – is usually known as postmodernism, literally, that which comes after modernism. In contrast to post-positivist critiques, postmodernism entails 'the revision not simply of hypotheses or even "paradigms", but of the modes of reasoning and logic once considered "natural" or imprescriptible'.[4]

To say that there is confusion surrounding the understanding of postmodernism would be a gross understatement; the main problem would seem to be that there are probably as many interpretations of postmodernism as there are postmodernists. Some writers have seen this as a wilful act, such that 'there seems to be an unwritten agreement among postmodernists that postmodernism should forever elude a consensus as to its definition'.[5] The philosopher Lawrence Cahoone likened postmodernism to a 'family of intellectual movements' whose members 'not only express conflicting views, but are interested in barely overlapping subject matters: art, communications media, history, economics, politics, ethics, cosmology, theology, methodology, literature, education.[6] Continuing the analogy, however, 'some of the most important members of the family refuse to be called by the family name. And there are distant relations who deny that they are related at all.'[7] Furthermore, the family resemblances between members overlap in the same way as they do in 'real' families. So, for example, postmodern architecture might share the same eye colour as postmodern philosophy, which might in turn share the same curly hair as postmodern literary theory. Thus, although architecture and literary theory might have no obvious common features, they are still recognizably related.

As we have seen, postmodernism refers, in the literal sense, to what comes *post* (after) the modern age; in other words, it is the age that follows modernism. Lyotard expressed this view as:

> The 'post-' of 'postmodern' has a sense of a simple succession, a diachronic sequence of periods in which each one is clearly identifiable. The 'post-' indicates something like a conversion: a new direction from a previous one.[8]

The difficulty with this interpretation is that what it defines is a period of time rather than an intellectual or artistic movement, since *whatever* movement followed the modern would be, in this literal sense, postmodern. Or, to put it another way, 'to say that the postmodern simply comes after the modern in diachronic succession is to say that it is the most recent modernism'.[9] Thus, since the postmodern age would, by definition, *succeed* the modern, there is little point in postmodernism bothering to critique modernism, because the latter would already be dead and buried.[10] As Lyotard again pointed out:

> I would argue that the project of modernity... has not been forsaken or forgotten but destroyed, 'liquidated'. There are several modes of destruction, several names which are symbols for them. 'Auschwitz' can be taken as a paradigmatic name for the tragic 'incompletion' of modernity.[11]

However, the modernists regard their movement as very much alive, and accuse postmodernism of wishing to 'get rid of the *uncompleted* [as they see it] project of modernism, that of the Enlightenment'.[12] Thus, as the social philosopher Jürgen Habermas argued:

> I think that instead of giving up modernity and its project as a lost cause, we should learn from the mistakes of those extravagant programs which have tried to negate modernity.[13]

The sociologist Anthony Giddens made a similar point. While he agreed with the postmodernists that we are living in an age in which

> sensory observation is permeated by theoretical categories, philosophical thought has in the main veered quite sharply away from empiricism... [and] we are much more clearly aware of the circularity of reason, as well as the problematic relations between knowledge and power[14]

he nevertheless maintained that this is merely 'modernity coming to understand itself' rather than the overcoming of modernity as such'.[15]

Furthermore, since the modern age can be characterized as the age of progress and invention, it is difficult to imagine what could possibly follow it. The end of the modernist age is, by definition, the end of the need for progress and thus, in a sense, a perfect state. Usher and Edwards (among others) have pointed out this 'double signification' of the word 'end' as meaning, at the same time, that modernism has achieved its goal (its end-point), and that it has thereby brought about its termination (ending).[16] This is partly the meaning of postmodernism taken by advocates of, for example, postmodern architecture, who can see no prospect of further development, only of a mixing and matching of past styles, what the American critic Fredric Jameson has termed 'pastiche'.[17] As Sarup pointed out, the practice of pastiche, 'the imitation of dead styles', suggests that:

> we are unable to focus on our present. We have lost our ability to locate ourselves historically. As a society we have become incapable of dealing with time.[18]

Thus, for Lyotard, 'postmodern architecture finds itself condemned to undertake a series of minor modifications in a space inherited from modernity'.[19] This notion of postmodernism as representing the end of progress is also the meaning usually taken by the writers of the growing number of books proclaiming the end of, among other things, economics, history, knowledge, politics (in its various guises) and the professions.[20]

A second interpretation of postmodernism is to contrast it with what is modern, that is, with what is currently in fashion, rather than with what is modern*ist*. This interpretation would suggest that ideas, movements, schools of art and so on become modern for a time before becoming *post*modern. However, in this sense, the term 'postmodern' is synonymous with old fashioned or with no longer being modern, and this clashes with the more usually understood meaning of the term as being, rather confusingly, *pre*modern or *avant garde*. Thus, as Lyotard pointed out, 'A work can become modern only if it is first postmodern. Postmodernism thus understood is not modernism at its end but in the nascent state.'[21]

However, Lyotard elsewhere retracted this meaning of postmodernism as *avant garde* or 'the latest thing' in favour of an epistemological meaning. 'Postmodern is not to be taken in a periodizing [that is, as initiating a new period of history] sense',[22] but rather as a *critique* of the modernist project. Thus:

> Postmodernity is not a new age, it is the rewriting of some features modernity had tried or pretended to gain, particularly in founding its legitimation upon the purpose of the general emancipation of mankind.[23]

Postmodernity, on this reading, has a critical relationship to modernity rather than a temporal one: it is 'in every respect parasitic on modernity; it lives and feeds on its achievements and on its dilemmas';[24] and 'postmodernity is modernity coming of age... looking at itself at a distance rather than from inside'.[25] Modernity and postmodernity can therefore exist side by side, although their relationship is somewhat fraught.

Probably the most straightforward definition of postmodernism as a critique of modernism is provided by Lyotard, who stated 'simplifying to the extreme, I define *postmodern* as incredulity toward metanarratives'.[26] We saw in the previous chapter that a metanarrative or grand narrative refers to an appeal to the legitimization of knowledge that lies outside the procedures for generating and/or disseminating that knowledge, or more simply, to an overarching philosophy that provides an explanation for a particular discipline or system of knowledge, but which does not itself require justification or proof. A metanarrative is thus the 'bottom line' of a discipline or discourse that is taken as an act of faith. The philosopher Richard Rorty referred to this stance as 'metaphysics', in which the metaphysician is someone who assumes that concepts such as justice, science, knowledge, faith, morality, philosophy and so on have a real essence.[27] Metaphysics therefore includes:

any such thought-system which depends on an unassailable foundation, a first principle or unimpeachable ground upon which a whole
hierarchy of meanings may be constructed.[28]

Thus, Marxists appeal to history as justification for their discourse,
humanists to 'human nature', and theologians to God or the Bible. The
modernist tradition of empirical science, however, sets its own grand
narrative apart from metaphysics, which it sees as lacking a firm foundation in reality (recall Hume's outburst against sophistry and illusion). Thus, for Wittgenstein, we should 'say nothing except what can
be said, that is propositions of natural science'.[29]

In contrast, the postmodernists place *all* grand narratives on the
same footing, that is, as equally deserving of an attitude of incredulity.
In the words of French philosopher Jacques Derrida, we live in a
'decentred universe' without recourse to a final and absolute authority.[30] From the postmodern perspective, the only difference between
modernism and all the other 'isms' is that Marxism, humanism,
Catholicism, Buddhism and so on are based on an irrational belief in
history, human nature, God and Buddha respectively, whereas modernism is based, ironically, on an irrational belief in rationality itself.[31]

Seen in this way, the principal achievement of the Enlightenment
was to replace religion with science as the dominant belief system; science, in a sense, *became* religion. Thus:

> Once upon a time we felt the need to worship something which lay
> beyond the visible world. Beginning in the seventeenth century we tried
> to substitute a love of truth for a love of God, treating the world
> described by science as a quasi divinity.[32]

The way in which Hume 'lost his faith' in the scientific method following his realization of the intractability of the problem of induction also
offers an interesting parallel with religion.

This is a particularly damaging critique, since it will be recalled that
those founders of modernism, the empiricists, spoke out with particular vehemence against so-called metaphysical philosophers such as
Kant and Descartes,[33] who believed that truth could be arrived at
through pure thought or introspection. However, according to the
above critique, 'although [the empiricists] were all hostile to "metaphysics" in the derogatory sense of extravagant system-building, they
were all, in the wider neutral sense, considerable metaphysicians in
their own right'.[34] Thus, from the postmodern perspective, the empiri
cists rejected all other metaphysical systems for the metaphysics of
experimental science and an appeal to the senses as the only way of
validating knowledge.

THE PROBLEM OF RELATIVISM

However, in asserting that *all* metanarratives, including that of science, should be looked upon with incredulity, postmodernism is opening itself to a charge of relativism; indeed, this is often seen as its distinguishing feature, such that 'much postmodern thought may be regarded as a somewhat abandoned celebration of relativism'.[35] The philosophical doctrine of relativism can be traced back at least to the time of Plato, and argues that there is no absolute authority on which to make judgements. Instead, any given thing 'is to me such as it appears to me, and is to you such as it appears to you'.[36] From the postmodernist perspective, however, the influence of relativism originates largely from the work of Friedrich Nietzsche, for whom 'there are no eternal facts, just as there are no absolute truths'.[37]

Nietzsche's rejection of absolute truths had at least two foundations. First, he argued for moral relativism on pragmatic grounds:

> For we have no organ at all for knowledge, for 'truth': we 'know' (or believe or imagine) precisely as much as may be useful in the interest of the human herd, the species: and even what is here called 'usefulness' is in the end only a belief, something imagined and perhaps precisely that most fatal piece of stupidity by which we shall one day perish.[38]

Knowledge, particularly moral knowledge, has its roots in what is useful to society: 'first of all, one calls individual actions good or bad quite irrespective of their motives but solely on account of their useful or harmful consequences'.[39] But 'soon, however, one forgets the origin of these designations and believes that the quality "good" and "evil" is inherent in the actions themselves'.[40] Thus, moral judgements are made initially according to ends rather than means: if an action has a beneficial outcome, it is judged to be good. Over time, however, the 'goodness' in these acts is attributed to the means by which the ends are arrived at. Finally:

> One goes further and accords the predicate good or evil no longer to the individual motive but to the whole nature of a man out of whom the motive grows as the plant does from the soil.[41]

The inevitable conclusion of this position is that when we judge an action to be good, we are, in fact, merely stating its usefulness: to say that honesty is a good thing is to say that for people to be honest is beneficial to society. Since, however, societies change over time and are different in different parts of the world, so too are conceptions of goodness different at different times and in different places. For Nietzsche, then, 'There are no moral phenomena at all, only a moral interpretation of phenomena.'[42]

The second foundation for Nietzsche's rejection of absolute truth is an argument from language that prefigures the work of Wittgenstein, the structuralists, the logical positivists and the postmodernist philosophers. Thus:

> mankind set up in language a separate world beside the other world, a place it took to be so firmly set that, standing upon it, it could lift the rest of the world off its hinges and make itself master of it.[43]

This is, in fact, the point that Foucault made almost a century later, that until the sixteenth century, language was inseparable from truth, indeed, that language *was* truth. The name 'horse' contained the essence of what it named; the word *was*, in some sense, the horse itself. Thus, for Nietzsche, '[man] really thought that in language he possessed knowledge of the world'.[44]

However, Nietzsche recognized this equivalence between language and reality to be a myth, such that 'all our words are based on equations between unequal things, and they can never have more than a tenuous relation to what they represent'.[45] It is, however, a comforting myth that holds society together, and, as such, society is prepared to deceive itself that it is the truth. Thus, 'Something will now be fixed that should from now on be "truth": what is invented, in other words, is a standardizing, valid and compulsory designation of things.'[46] Ultimately, however, language cannot define what is true:

> So what is truth? A mobile army of metaphors, metonyms, anthropomorphisms – in short an aggregate of human relationships which, poetically and rhetorically heightened, become transposed and elaborated, and which, after popular usage, pose as fixed, canonical, obligatory. Truths are illusions whose illusoriness is overlooked.[47]

This extreme relativist position results in two difficulties: first, it often evokes a moral or aesthetic repugnance, and second, it is logically and epistemologically inconsistent.

The repugnance with which many people regard relativism stems from its 'anything goes' image, such that 'the fear of "anything goes", of chaos of (in)difference, arises in the context of an apparent loss of the prospect of order, certainty and security'.[48] This fear of relativism can provoke extreme reactions in some writers, leading to personal attacks on its alleged perpetrators. Thus, for the historian Felipe Fernández-Armesto, Nietzsche was 'a sexually inexperienced invalid' whose 'repulsive doctrines' were 'a morbid fantasy, warped and man-gled out of his own lonely, sickly self-hatred'.[49] Similarly, Kierkegaard's 'inclinations were idle and selfish' and he 'found it easier to feel shame than to act honourably',[50] Schopenhauer espoused a nihilism that 'is only advocated by the embittered and the failed',[51] and Richard Rorty, one of today's leading pragmatist philosophers, 'belongs by self-ascription to the community of conventionally liberal, politically correct, secularist professors' whose '"pragmatism" amounts to a preference for his own inclinations'.[52] As for relativism itself, it will lead to a situation in which 'liars will have nothing to prove – and defenders of truth will have no case to demand of them'.[53]

Whereas Fernández-Armesto condemned all relativists together, along with their 'repulsive doctrines', it might be useful to distinguish between a number of different forms of relativism. In the realm of aes-thetics, relativism can lead to value assertions such as 'the Spice Girls are better than Bach' (or vice versa), with no recourse to a higher authority to make a definitive judgement; in the realm of epistemolo-gy, it requires us to give the same consideration to creation myths[54] as we give to Darwinian evolutionism; and in the realm of ethics, we are forced to accept the moral perspective of the pornographer or of the murderer as having an equal footing with that of the priest. There is no absolute right and wrong; instead, 'man is the measure of all things'.[55]

While aesthetic relativism can be rather irritating, especially to the proponents of 'high' culture ('high', of course, being an absolutist term: for the relativist, there is no high or low), epistemological and moral relativism are not only annoying, but also rather dangerous. For example, the feminist writer Stevi Jackson[56] asks how, from a relativist perspective, we are to judge between the rape victim's account of forced sexual intercourse and the rapist's account of pleasurable seduction. Similarly, Alison Assiter has asserted that 'in a world in which there are horrendous wars taking place, the environment is being destroyed, and there is mass starvation, this [relativist] view is morally and politically reprehensible'.[57] However, the argument that relativism is dangerous or that it can lead to the justification of unpleasant, illegal or even downright evil practices has no *logical* standing, since to the relativist, what is unpleasant, illegal and evil is itself open to individual judgement and opinion.

A second and stronger critique of relativism comes from turning its own arguments back on itself.[58] If no doctrine can be shown to be absolutely true, the doctrine of relativism also cannot be shown to be true. Thus, if I espouse the doctrine of relativism, I have to allow that others, from their relative perspective, have equal grounds for rejecting it. If relativism is true, it is, by its own admission, also not true. As Roger Scruton pointed out, 'The man who tells you truth does not exist is asking you not to believe him. So don't.'[59]

These objections to the doctrine of relativism have also been used against postmodernism, since, as we saw earlier, postmodernism would appear to be rooted in relativism. However, I believe that this perception underlies an essential misunderstanding of the postmodernist position. If it *is* a relativist philosophy, it is based on a peculiar kind of relativism (which some would argue is not relativism at all), and in order fully to understand it and its implications, we must look in some detail at the origins of postmodernism.

A SHORT HISTORY OF POSTMODERNISM

The philosopher Lawrence Cahoone has traced the usage of the term 'postmodernism' (or, as it is sometimes written, 'post-modernism') back almost one hundred years.[60] Thus, it was first employed by the German philosopher Rudolph Pannwitz in 1917 to describe, appropriately enough, Nietzsche's notion of the nihilism of the early twentieth century. Cahoone then traces its appearances in literature, theology, social history and architecture, before it emerges as a philosophical movement in the 1980s. For the purposes of this book, it is the philosophical strand of postmodernism on which I intend to focus.

Saussure, Barthes and structuralism

Rather ironically, postmodern philosophy has its roots in the attempt by modernism to extend its influence into areas that are, arguably, beyond the scope of rational scientific thought, namely language and literature. This attempt to apply the methods of science to the study of language was initiated in the early years of the twentieth century by the Swiss linguist Ferdinand de Saussure, who was particularly interested in semiotics or the science of signs. For Saussure, a sign comprised two components – a *signifier* (a spoken or written word) and a *signified* (the concept or meaning of that word) – and this sign has as its *referent* something in the world. Thus, the word 'book' *signifies* the concept of a bound collection of paper pages, which in turn *refers* to the object from which you are now reading, which is the referent of the sign.

This much, of course, is fairly straightforward, but Saussure's ground-breaking (if, in retrospect, fairly obvious) observation was that there is no necessary relationship between the signifier (the word) and the signified (the concept). There is no reason why we should use the word 'book' to signify the concept of a bound collection of paper pages, any more than the French use the word '*livre*'; the relationship between the word and the concept to which it refers is purely arbitrary. Similarly, the relationship between the whole sign (the signifier and the signified together) and its referent in the world is also arbitrary. There is no ontological reason why the word 'book' should be associated with the object you are reading; the word takes its meaning not from its referent, but instead from other words. Thus, 'book' has no intrinsic meaning, but is differentiated by its relationship to similar words such as 'look' and 'boot'. Similarly, the *concept* of a book is differentiated by its relationship to similar concepts such as pamphlet and journal. We could equally use the word 'splot' to refer to a bound collection of paper pages, so long as 'splot' is sufficiently different from all other words in the language. As Saussure put it, 'in the linguistic system, there are only differences'.[61]

This position on the structure of language is, of course, a form of relativism, since Saussure is claiming that words and signs only have meaning in relation to other words and signs; the word 'book' has meaning because it is different from the words 'look' and 'boot'. However, although this form of relativism is fairly innocuous, it was the application of semiotics to literature and, significantly, to the wider cultural world by the structuralists that posed the first real challenge to the metanarrative of scientific empiricism.

One of the leading exponents of structuralism was the French literary critic Roland Barthes, who applied the science of semiotics to literature[62] as well as to fields as diverse as wrestling, the Citroën car and an image of Greta Garbo.[63] Structuralism was influential in two ways: first, it provided an objective method for the analysis of literature, which 'like any other product of language, is a *construct*, whose mechanisms could be classified and analysed like the objects of any other science';[64] and second, it made a strong link between literary criticism and the broader field of cultural studies, paving the way, as we shall see, for postmodernism.

However, there is clearly an internal conflict in a critical method that, at the same time, sees its object of study as a subjective construct and itself as an objective science. This inconsistency was highlighted by Barthes in his 1968 essay 'The death of the author',[65] in which he rejected the notion of 'the voice of a single person, the *author* "confiding" in us'.[66] The aim of literary criticism was therefore no longer an attempt to arrive at the 'true' meaning of the text as intended by the author:

> Once the author is removed, the claim to decipher a text becomes quite futile. To give a text an Author is to impose a limit on that text, to furnish it with a final signified, to close the writing.[67]

Because of the arbitrary relationship between the signifier, the signified and their referent in the world, any attempt to understand the meaning of a text as it was intended by its author is not only impossible, but also imposes a limit on what that text might 'say' to the reader, who, Barthes claimed, is the real creative force in literature. The reader, then, is 'that *someone* who holds together in a single field all the traces by which the written text is constituted', and 'the birth of the reader must be at the cost of the death of the Author'.[68]

Derrida and post-structuralism

Eventually, this constructivist (or perhaps we should say 'deconstructivist') tendency of structuralism overcame its scientific roots to produce a *post-structuralism* in which each reader provided her own interpretation (her own reading,[69] that is, *deconstructing* the text and thereby recreating it for herself. Deconstructionism, then, rebuilds at the same time as it takes apart. It is:

> not synonymous with 'destruction'. It is in fact much closer to the original meaning of the word 'analysis', which etymologically means 'to undo'... The deconstruction of a text does not proceed by random doubt or arbitrary subversion, but by the careful teasing out of warring forces of signification within the text.[70]

The above quotation appears to suggest that there is a method associated with deconstruction, although Barthes' later writing to some extent refutes this.[71] Thus:

> *at a certain moment*, therefore, it is necessary to turn against Method, or at least to treat it without any founding privilege as one of the voices of plurality – as a *view*, a spectacle mounted in the text, the text which all in all is the only 'true' result of any research.[72]

Method is unnecessary because, in any text, there is a conflict between what the author wishes to say and what it is possible to express in language. Writing can never fully convey the true meaning intended by the

writer, and all texts therefore contain 'gaps' or *aporias* that are waiting
to be filled by the reader. Thus, 'a deconstructive reading attends to the
deconstructive process *always* occurring in texts and *already* there
waiting to be read'.[73]

Barthes was first and foremost a literary critic, but it was Jacques
Derrida who pushed post-structuralism out beyond its origins in the
study of literature towards a position on the world in general, and
hence to be a challenge to science. As we have seen, Derrida wrote of a
'decentred' universe devoid of certainties, and also famously proclaimed that 'there is nothing outside of the text';[74] in other words, the
whole world was a potential subject for analysis by deconstruction. To
understand what Derrida meant by these statements, we have to
understand that by 'writing', he meant not only the inscription of
words or symbols on a page, but also cinematography, choreography,
painting, music, sculpture, sport, politics, cybernetics and life itself.[75]
Thus, a text (what is written) also takes on an extended form as a
shorthand for *all* attempts at representation. To deconstruct a text,
then, is to tease out the multiple and often contradictory meanings
(the gaps or *aporias*) that are inherent in all representations of the
world. Whenever a text (in Derrida's broad sense of the word) is decon-
structed, it therefore results *not* in a clearer understanding of the
author's intentions, but in another text, another representation (what
he refers to as a supplement), which is itself open to being decon-
structed. Thus:

> Through this sequence of supplements a necessity is announced: that
> of an infinite chain, ineluctably multiplying the supplementary media-
> tions that produce the sense of the very thing they defer.[76]

Gayatri Chakravorty Spivak (Derrida's translator) called this the 'fall
into the abyss of deconstruction', in which 'a further deconstruction
deconstructs deconstruction' and so on *ad infinitum* in 'the pleasure of
the bottomless'.[77]

We can see, then, that for Derrida, the aim of critical (deconstructive) writing was not a narrowing down towards a single truth, but
rather a broadening out towards multiple truths, another link in
the 'infinite chain' of supplements. The more a text is analysed, the
more it is decentred by the production of supplementary texts. All
that lies outside the text is more texts: there is, then, *nothing* outside
the text(s).

But Derrida did not merely write *about* post-structuralism, he *wrote*
post-structuralism; that is, he simply wrote. For Derrida, as we have
seen, the aim of writing was an attempt not to get closer to a single

truth, but to challenge that very idea. Thus, 'writing (and the written text) is itself the message rather than merely conveying the message'.[78] Through the use of puns, wordplays and general jokiness, where the text is subject to 'drift' with no obvious starting point and no clear goal, Derrida encourages us:

> to get out of a habit of mind which sees the only point of reading a text to be that of extracting knowledge and truth which is relevant, useful and efficatious. In other words, we have to start undoing the presuppositions and predispositions which hold us captive.[79]

We do not read in order to discover the truth; instead, reading is the starting point for our own writing, our own construction of our own text.

Lyotard and postmodernism

Derrida's assertion that the entire world could be 'read' as if it were a text, along with his 'playful' approach to writing, was an early indication of what was later to come to be known as the postmodern stance.[80] However, it was not until the publication of Jean-François Lyotard's book *The Postmodern Condition: A Report on Knowledge*[81] in 1979 that the term 'postmodernism' was first consciously employed in a philosophical sense.[82] As its title suggests, Lyotard adopted an epistemological approach to postmodernism, and as Jameson pointed out in the Foreword to the English edition, it presented a 'discussion of the consequences of the new views of scientific research and its paradigms, opened up by theorists like Thomas Kuhn and Paul Feyerabend'.[83]

However, Lyotard's work opened the floodgates to a host of self-styled postmodern artists, novelists and architects who seized on the perceived 'anything goes' message of deconstructionism, often to disguise their own lack of imagination. Architecture, in particular, has suffered at the hand of a relativist perspective in which all styles and periods are considered equal, and all are fair game for a 'mix and match' approach to design that can be seen in many of our newer public buildings and shopping centres. Also, because architecture is the most publicly visible of the arts, postmodernism has become associated in the public imagination with eclecticism and, ultimately, relativism.

Lyotard, however, rejected this eclectic approach as junk postmodernism:

Eclecticism is the degree zero of contemporary general culture: you listen to reggae, you watch a western, you eat McDonald's at midday and local cuisine at night, you wear Paris perfume in Tokyo and dress retro in Hong Kong, knowledge is the stuff of TV game shows.[84]

But if this popular conception is a false postmodernism, what is the 'real' postmodernism? Indeed, does it make any sense to talk of reality from a postmodern perspective, or are we, as Jean Baudrillard suggested, living in an age of 'hyperreality'[85] brought about by the pervasion into our lives of images from film, television and advertising, so that we can no longer tell reality from illusion?

For Lyotard, 'real' postmodernism is, confusingly, concerned with the very issue of how we can identify what 'real' postmodernism really is, that is, with the question of legitimation, and in particular, with the legitimation of knowledge. Thus, for Lyotard, it is not a question of what is real and what is not, or even of what counts as knowledge and what does not, but rather of how those decisions are made and who makes them. Thus:

> Take any civil law as an example: it states that a given category of citizens must perform a specific kind of action. Legitimation is the process by which a legislator is authorized to promulgate such a law as a norm. Now take the example of a scientific statement: it is subject to the rule that a statement must fulfill a given set of conditions in order to be accepted as scientific. In this case, legitimation is the process by which a 'legislator' dealing with scientific discourse is authorized to prescribe the stated conditions (in general, conditions of internal consistency and experimental verification) determining whether a statement is to be included in that discourse for consideration by the scientific community.[86]

Similarly for Foucault:

> Each society has its own regime of truth, its 'general politics' of truth: that is, the types of discourse which it accepts and makes function as true; the mechanisms and instances which enable one to distinguish true and false statements, the means by which each is sanctified; the techniques and procedures accorded value in the acquisition of truth; the status of those who are charged with saying what counts as true.[87]

From a postmodernist perspective, it is not a case of 'anything goes'; postmodernists are not, contrary to the general view, claiming that there is no difference between the Spice Girls and Bach, or between classical Greek architecture and modernist high-rise tower blocks. Instead, they are pointing out that of course there are differences (to reiterate the claim made by Saussure, 'there are *only* differences'), but that the crucial question to be asked is not 'What are those differences?', but 'Who decides on them?' In other words, it is a question of legitimation, and as Lyotard went on to add, 'knowledge and power are simply two sides of the same question: who decides what knowledge is, and who knows what needs to be decided?'[88]

RELATIVISM REVISITED

To return to the original issue of relativism, the absolutist would argue that the question: 'Is Bach better than the Spice Girls?' is a valid question which can be answered by consulting an expert, that is, by an appeal to authority; the relativist would claim that the question has no meaning, and that we have no grounds for making such a judgement; and the postmodernist would claim that while it is a valid question, the answer we get depends on who we ask, and that a better question would be: 'Who decides whether Bach is better than the Spice Girls, and from where does she get the power and authority to make such a decision?'

This interpretation of the postmodern position on relativism can be defended, following Bhaskar,[89] by making the distinction between epistemic and judgemental relativism (or, as Bhaskar refers to it, 'relativity'). Epistemic relativism, to which all postmodernists would subscribe, argues that knowledge is socially constructed and that we can have no access to a realm of 'pure' or absolute knowledge. Judgemental relativism, which some 'classical' postmodernists would accept, but which I (along with Bhaskar) would wish to reject, makes the further claim that, because all forms of knowledge are social constructs, we are therefore unable to compare and discriminate between them.

In fact, the postmodern position that I am advocating here is in many ways similar to Bhaskar's own project of transcendental realism.[90] Like postmodernism, transcendental realism is critical of the monistic and deductive aspects of positivism; like postmodernism, it argues that 'all beliefs are socially produced, so that all knowledge is transient';[91] like postmodernism, it claims that social phenomena have to be interpreted or 'read'; like postmodernism, it sees knowledge as largely inseparable from language; but *unlike* postmodernism, it 'embraces a coherent account of the nature of nature, society, human agency and philosophy (including itself)'.[92]

It also, by its own account, has a different agenda from postmodernism, being concerned with ontology, the nature of being, rather than with epistemology, the nature of knowledge. For the transcendental realists, the philosophy of science must have an ontological foundation, since we cannot talk about knowledge without first examining what there is to be known. For the postmodernists, this is not a major concern, because knowledge exists as an object of study independent of any external reality. To borrow the words of Wittgenstein, the postmodernists are interested in 'only the network and not what the network describes'.[93] Thus, whereas a number of postmodern philosophers hold that reality itself is a social construct (as opposed to knowledge about reality), Bhaskar makes the ontological realist claim that reality exists independent of human beings. For Bhaskar, then:

> a realist position in the philosophy of science will be a theory about the nature of the being, not the knowledge, of the objects investigated by science – roughly that they exist, and act independently of human activity, and hence of both sense-experience and thought.[94]

It is, however, possible to hold a postmodern stance on epistemology while agreeing with Bhaskar's transcendental realist ontology. For example, the postmodernist philosopher Richard Rorty does not believe that reality is socially constructed. Indeed, he specifically states that:

> To say that the world is out there, that it is not our creation, is to say, with common sense, that most things in space and time are the effects of causes which do not include human mental states.[95]

More specifically, 'the world is out there, but descriptions of the world are not'.[96]

Although Rorty is often described as an anti-realist, he claimed that he wished to construct 'a position which is beyond realism and antirealism'.[97] In fact, Rorty takes a pragmatist and self-confessed ethnocentric view in which 'there is nothing to be said about either truth or rationality apart from descriptions of the familiar procedures of justification which a given society – *ours* – uses in one or other area of inquiry'.[98] Thus, in structuralist terminology, the sign 'true' means the same in all cultures, just as signs such as 'here' and 'me' mean the same, although the referent of the sign will, of course, be different. When you and I both use the word 'me', we use it in the same way, although the person I am referring to is different from the person you are referring to. Similarly, when we both use the word 'true', we use it in the same way, although not necessarily to describe the same things; furthermore, our descriptions might well be contradictory.

It is clear, then, that both Rorty and Bhaskar support epistemic relativism, but would wish to argue (albeit for different reasons) that it is possible to judge between different truth claims. Thus, Bhaskar would judge a truth claim with reference to a transcendent 'real' world, whereas Rorty would judge it according to the 'ethnocentric' criteria of his own culture. Discriminations and comparisons clearly *are* made, and the interesting questions are concerned with who makes these discriminations and how they are made. Furthermore, this position of accepting epistemic relativism but rejecting judgemental relativism is reasonable and logically coherent, since, as Brown pointed out, 'assertions of *judgemental* relativism are not in the least entailed by the position of *epistemological* relativism. Indeed, in some ways, the two are opposite'.[99] Thus, it is logically possible to assert, at the same time, that two statements are both based on socially constructed knowledge, but that one is preferable to the other. As Smart pointed out, 'if, under conditions of postmodernity anything may go, it is not the case that any, or every thing does go, has to go, or has to be accepted'.[100]

I hope that I have now legitimated my own claims that postmodernism does not necessarily entail an extreme judgemental relativism, that it is possible to make value judgements from a position of knowledge, and that the most important epistemological questions are not concerned with the foundations of knowledge, but with the power to legitimate knowledge, that is, to define what counts as knowledge and what does not. For some postmodernists, then, knowledge (and hence what we accept as truth) is not so much socially constructed as socially validated. The relationship between relativism and postmodernism will be explored further in the following chapter. However, for now, Lyotard's 'incredulity towards metanarratives', which I took as the defining feature of postmodernism, can be seen not as a relativist *rejection* of metanarratives (including the metanarrative of science), but as a stance of uncertainty; Lyotard is questioning not so much their truth claims as the authority by which they make truth claims.

Postmodernism, at least on this reading, is therefore concerned not directly with knowledge (that is, with epistemological questions), but with power (that is, with political questions) and the struggle to define and impose truth.[101] In particular, it challenges the metanarrative of science as being somehow superior to other metanarratives such as Marxism, humanism, Catholicism and Buddhism, a position that has been summarized as: 'there is no *one* story, although there is *a* story [the Enlightenment narrative of science], a very powerful story, that says there is'.[102] Thus, postmodernism is not arguing *against* empirical science, but instead against its privileged position as the 'one story', the only valid way of distinguishing what is true from what is false, and more importantly, what is truth from what is falsity.[103] In a sense, then, the postmodernist position is challenging the very *idea* of truth as it is generally conceived in Western industrial society.

THE END OF POSTMODERNISM?

As we have already seen, this challenge to the absolutist notion of truth has been attacked by a number of critics of postmodernism. Felipe Fernández-Armesto, it will be recalled, attempted to defend the idea of truth itself from the 'repulsive doctrine' of relativism, whereas other writers wished to uphold the truth-value of their particular project, whether it be Marxism, feminism or any other 'ism'. The most damaging critique of postmodernism in recent years has probably come, ironically, from a book that makes no real claim to rebut postmodernism at all. The book, entitled *Intellectual Impostures*,[104] by the scientists Alan Sokal and Jean Bricmont, was hailed on its publication in 1997 as the nemesis of postmodernism, and reportedly 'sent shock waves through the [French] Left Bank establishment',[105] to the extent that even normally liberal and objective publications such as the *Guardian* newspaper claimed that the book demonstrated that 'modern French philosophy is a load of old tosh'.[106]

Unfortunately, the book's reputation has gone very much before it, and anyone who claims, as Jon Henly did in the *Guardian*, that it shows postmodernism to be 'a load of old tosh', has clearly not read it. If they had, they would have noted on the first page of the Preface that its authors make a far more modest claim for their project. The book was written in the wake of a now famous 'spoof' article by Alan Sokal[107] as a critique of the way in which certain French writers had abused scientific concepts in their work. Thus, they write in the Preface:

> famous intellectuals such as Lacan, Kristeva, Irigaray, Baudrillard and Deleuze have repeatedly abused scientific concepts and terminology... We make no claim that this invalidates the rest of their work, on which we suspend judgement.[108]

This claim is repeated more overtly at the start of Chapter 1, where:

> We make no claim to analyse postmodernist thought in general; rather, our aim is to draw attention to a relatively little-known aspect, namely the repeated abuse of concepts and terminology coming from mathematics and physics.[109]

Again, several pages later:

> we do not purport to judge Lacan's psychoanalysis, Deleuze's philosophy or Latour's concrete work in sociology. We limit ourselves to their statements about the mathematical and physical sciences or about elementary problems in the philosophy of science.[110]

It might appear that I am overstating the case, but this book is cited by almost every critic of postmodernism as being a devastating refutation of the whole of contemporary French thought. It is thus important to point out that anyone who bothered to read beyond the sensationalist quotations on the back cover, even if only as far as page 11, would have encountered at least three clear statements of the authors' intentions. And these intentions are modest: they claim merely to critique certain passages in the writing of certain French philosophers that deal with an abuse of scientific terms and concepts, and 'it goes without saying that we are not competent to judge the non-scientific aspects of these authors' work'.[111] However, as well as not claiming to critique postmodern*ism*, neither are they claiming to critique postmodern*ists*. Thus:

> It is true that the French authors discussed in this book do not all regard themselves as 'postmodernist' or 'poststructuralist'. Some of these texts were published prior to the emergence of these intellectual currents, and some of these authors reject any link with these currents.[112]

They continue: 'We do not want to get involved in terminological disputes about the distinctions between "postmodernism", "poststructuralism" and so forth', and add that 'the validity or invalidity of our arguments can in no way depend on the use of a word'.[113] Perhaps not, but the *application* of those arguments to a critique of postmodernism clearly depends on the use of the word 'postmodernism'.

They further acknowledge that many other writers who have no connection whatsoever with postmodernism have abused scientific concepts in similar ways, and that:

> these include virtually all applications of mathematics to the social sciences (for example economics), physicists' speculations in popular books (for example Hawking, Penrose), sociobiology, cognitive science, information theory, the Copenhagen interpretation of quantum mechanics, and the use of scientific concepts and formulae by Hume, La Mettrie, D'Holbach, Helvetius, Condillac, Comte, Durkheim, Pareto, Engels and sundry others.[114]

So how did the authors come to choose a handful of contemporary French writers from among this very distinguished company?: 'Quite simply, Sokal stumbled on most of these texts in the course of writing his parody, and we decided, after reflection, that it was worth making them public.'[115] Compared to the enormous hype surrounding this book, its 'devastating critique of some of France's best-known thinkers'[116] hardly amounts to any sort of critique of postmodernism as a branch of philosophical thought.

The book, however, has a second aim, a 'critique of epistemic relativism',[117] which is, if anything, even less devastating than its critique of postmodernism (although, rather predictably, the two are conflated to refer to more or less the same project). Sokal and Bricmont begin by noting the enormity of their undertaking: 'We are aware that we will be dealing with difficult problems concerning the nature of knowledge and objectivity, which have worried philosophers for centuries',[118] and acknowledge that 'we are well aware that we will be criticized for our lack of formal philosophical training',[119] later commenting that 'it goes without saying that we claim no special competence in history, sociology or politics'.[120] Nevertheless, 'this sort of objection leaves us cold [and] seems particularly irrelevant here'.[121]

Having spent so much effort decrying relativism, it is rather ironic that they do not spot their own interdisciplinary relativist stance. For example, they accuse their targeted French philosophers of 'a self-assurance that far outstrips their scientific competence',[122] since 'many concepts used by scientists... contain hidden ambiguities'.[123] Thus:

> In order to address these subjects meaningfully, one has to understand the relevant scientific theories at a rather deep and inevitably technical level; a vague understanding, at the level of popularizations, won't suffice.[124]

However, when it comes to addressing the subject of philosophy, the same rules simply do not apply. Sokal and Bricmont, who freely admit that 'neither of us holds a diploma in philosophy', [125] appear to be totally undaunted by what they themselves have identified as the 'difficult problems concerning the nature of knowledge and objectivity which have worried philosophers for centuries'. Furthermore, after claiming to be concerned only with the misuse of scientific terminology by certain French writers, a task for which they are eminently qualified, they now turn their attention to 'certain intellectual aspects of postmodernism that have had an impact on the humanities and the social sciences',[126] a task for which they are the first to admit that they are eminently *not* qualified. Thus, after stating at the outset of their book that they make no claim to analyse postmodernist thought in general, they nevertheless make a half-hearted and ill-informed attempt at a philosophical critique of relativism (which they erroneously take to be interchangeable with postmodernism) and arrive at the (hardly original) conclusion that:

> Postmodernism has three principal negative effects: a waste of time in the human sciences, a cultural confusion that favors obscurantism, and a weakening of the political left.[127]

It is this final objection of a weakening of the political left, or more generally of a denial of the possibility of political commitment, that has done most harm to the postmodern movement. The objection is usually associated with the relativist stance of postmodernism, and asks how a commitment to *any* cause is possible if there are no grand narratives to underpin belief. I have already begun to explore a form of postmodern thought that accepts on the one hand that there are no grand narratives, but on the other that it is still possible to make informed choices. In the next chapter, I shall develop that argument further to look beyond the 'classic' formulation of postmodernism, and to explore how it might be possible to make knowledge-claims in a world without certainties.

NOTES

1. Blake, W. *The Marriage of Heaven and Hell*, 1793.
2. Kuhn, T.S. Reflections on my critics. In I. Lakatos and A. Musgrave (eds) *Criticism and the Growth of Knowledge*, Cambridge: Cambridge University Press, 1970, pp. 231–78.
3. Lyotard, J.-F. (1979) *The Postmodern Condition: A Report on Knowledge*, Manchester: Manchester University Press, 1984, pp. xxiii–xxiv. That is not to say that Lyotard is opposed to universal peace, but only to science as the means of achieving it.
4. Lyotard, J.-F. (1985) Ticket for a new stage. In J.-F. Lyotard *The Postmodern Explained to Children*, London: Turnaround, 1992, p. 99.
5. Simons, H.W. and Billig, M. *After Postmodernism*, London: Sage, 1994, p. 5.
6. Cahoone, L. *From Modernism to Postmodernism: An Anthology*, Malden, MA: Blackwell, 1996, p. 1.
7. *Ibid.*, p. 1.
8. Lyotard, J.-F. (1985) Note on the meaning of 'post-'. In J.-F. Lyotard *The Postmodern Explained to Children*, London: Turnaround, 1992, p. 90. Lyotard was not advocating this view, but pointing it out as a 'false' postmodernism.
9. Readings, B. *Introducing Lyotard*, London: Routledge, 1991, p. 54.
10. Although it is worth reading what Arthur Koestler has to say in his paper

'On not flogging dead horses', the problem is that you can never be quite sure that seemingly dead horses really are dead, so it is always worth giving them an extra kick, just to be sure. See Koestler, A. (1967) *The Ghost in the Machine*, London: Pan, 1971, pp. 391–5.

11. Lyotard, J.-F. (1984) Apostil on narratives. In J.-F. Lyotard *The Postmodern Explained to Children*, London: Turnaround, 1992, p. 30.

12. Lyotard, J.-F. (1982) Answering the question: what is postmodernism? In J.-F. Lyotard *The Postmodern Condition: A Report on Knowledge*, Manchester: Manchester University Press, 1984, p. 72. emphasis added. Lyotard is here referring to the work of Jürgen Habermas, in particular to his paper 'Modernity – an incomplete project' (see below).

13. Habermas, J. Modernity – an incomplete project, *New German Critique*, 1981, **22**, 3–15. These 'extravagant programs' were, of course, those of the postmodernists, whom Habermas described (much to their annoyance) as 'young conservatives'.

14. Giddens, A. *The Consequences of Modernity*, Cambridge: Polity Press, 1990, p. 49.

15. *Ibid.*, p. 48.

16. Usher, R. and Edwards R. *Postmodernism and Education*, London: Routledge, 1994, pp. 130–1.

17. Jameson, F. Postmodernism, or the cultural logic of capital, *New Left Review*, 1984, **146**, pp. 53–92.

18. Sarup, M. *An Introductory Guide to Post-structuralism and Postmodernism*, New York: Harvester Wheatsheaf, 1988, p. 133.

19. Lyotard, J.-F. (1985) Note on the meaning of 'post-'. In J.-F. Lyotard *The Postmodern Explained to Children*, London: Turnaround, 1992, p. 89.

20. At the last count (June 1998) there were over thirty such titles, ranging from the end of time and the end of the world to the end of 'isms'.

21. Lyotard, *op. cit.*, (1985), p. 79.

22. Lyotard, J.-F. and Thébaud, J.-L. *Just Gaming*, Minneapolis: University of Minnesota Press, 1979, p. 16.

23. Lyotard, J.-F. Rewriting modernity, *SubStance*, 1987, **54**, 8–9.

24. Heller, A. and Feher, F. *The Postmodern Political Condition*, Cambridge: Polity Press, 1988, pp. 10–11.

25. Bauman, Z. *Modernity and Ambivalence*, Cambridge: Polity Press, 1991, p. 272. This notion of postmodernism as 'modernity coming of age' is reminiscent of Giddens' earlier argument *against* postmodernism.

26. Lyotard, J.-F. (1979) *The Postmodern Condition: A Report on Knowledge*, Manchester: Manchester University Press, 1984, p. xxiv.

27. Rorty, R. *Contingency, Irony, and Solidarity*, Cambridge: Cambridge University Press, 1989, p. 74.

28. Eagleton, T. *Literary Theory*, Oxford: Blackwell, 1983, p. 132.

29. Wittgenstein, L. (1922) *Tractatus Logico-Philosophicus*, London: Routledge & Kegan Paul, 1971, 6.522. This is an expression of Wittgenstein's early 'logical positivist' position, and stands in direct contrast to his later views, which are discussed in Chapter 3.

30. Derrida, J. (1967) *Of Grammatology*, G.C. Spivak (trans.), Baltimore: John Hopkins University Press, 1974.
31. Paul Ricoeur has referred to this sceptical stance as 'the hermeneutics of suspicion'. See Ricoeur, P. *Lectures on Ideology and Utopia*, G.H. Taylor (ed.), New York: Columbia University Press, 1986.
32. Rorty, *op. cit.*, p. 22.
33. In fact, neither Kant nor Descartes were opposed to scientific empiricism, but instead saw metaphysics as the foundation of science (Descartes) or as a science in itself (Kant), a notion that, naturally, infuriated the empiricists. Thus, for Descartes, what we perceive with our senses must be true because God would not (indeed, could not) deceive us, while for Kant, metaphysics was 'the system of pure reason, that is, the *science* which exhibits in systematic connection the whole body (true as well as illusory) of philosophical knowledge arising out of pure reason': Kant, I. (1781) *The Critique of Pure Reason*, N. Kemp Smith (trans.), London: St Martin's Press, 1978, p. 869, emphasis added.
34. Midgely, M. *Wisdom, Information, and Wonder*, London: Routledge, 1991, p. 199.
35. Blackburn, S. *The Oxford Dictionary of Philosophy*, Oxford: Oxford University Press, 1994, p. 326.
36. This statement is ascribed to Protagoras in Plato's *Theatetus*, which can be found in Hamilton, E. and Cairns, H. *The Collected Dialogues of Plato*, Princeton, NJ: Princeton University, 1961, pp. 845–919.
37. Nietzsche, F. (1878) Human, all too human. In R.J. Hollingdale (ed.) *A Nietzsche Reader*, Harmondsworth: Penguin, 1977, p. 29.
38. Nietzsche, F. (1887) *The Gay Science*, 2nd edn, New York: Random House, 1974, p. 354.
39. Nietzsche, F. (1878) *op. cit.*, p. 71. Compare this with the pragmatist position described in Chapter 1.
40. *Ibid.*, p. 71.
41. *Ibid.*, p. 71.
42. Nietzsche, F. (1886) *Beyond Good and Evil*, Harmondsworth: Penguin, 1973, p. 108.
43. Nietzsche, F. (1878) *op. cit.*, p. 55.
44. *Ibid.*, p. 55.
45. Nietzsche, F. (1873) On truth and falsehood in an extra-moral sense. Cited in R. Hayman *Nietzsche*, London: Phoenix, 1997, p. 20.
46. *Ibid.*, p. 21.
47. *Ibid.*, pp. 21–2.
48. Smart, B. *Postmodernity*, London: Routledge, 1993, p. 103.
49. Fernández-Armesto, F. *Truth: A History*, London: Bantam Press, 1997, pp. 176–7.
50. *Ibid.*, p. 180.
51. *Ibid.*, p. 176.
52. *Ibid.*, p. 181.
53. *Ibid.*, p. 194.

54. Sorell, *op. cit.*, pointed out that some American Christian fundamentalist groups have taken to using the term 'creation *science*' in an attempt to give their ideas greater credibility.

55. Protagoras, *op. cit.*

56. Jackson, S. The amazing deconstructing woman, *Trouble and Strife*, 1992, **25**, 25–31.

57. Assiter, A. *Enlightened Women: Modernist Feminism in a Postmodern Age*, London: Routledge, 1996, p. 6.

58. This is known as the argument of self-referential incoherence, and can be found in Siegel, H. *Relativism Refuted: A Critique of Contemporary Epistemological Relativism*, Dordrecht: Reidel, 1987.

59. Scruton, R. *Modern Philosophy*, London: Arrow, 1994, p. 100.

60. Cahoone, *op. cit.*, p. 3.

61. Saussure, F. de (1916) *Course in General Linguistics*, London: Duckworth, 1983, p. 118.

62. See, for example, Barthes, R. (1966) Introduction to the structural analysis of narratives. In R. Barthes *Image Music Text*, S. Heath (trans.), London: Fontana, 1977, pp. 79–124; and also Barthes, R. (1970) *S/Z*, London: Cape, 1975, in which he spectacularly applies a structural analysis to Balzac's short story *Sarrasine*.

63. Barthes, R. (1957) *Mythologies*, New York: Hill & Wang, 1972.

64. Eagleton, *op. cit.*, p. 106.

65. Barthes, R. (1968) The death of the author. In R. Barthes *Image Music Text*, S. Heath (trans.), London: Fontana, 1977, pp. 142–8.

66. *Ibid.*, p. 143.

67. *Ibid.*, p. 147.

68. *Ibid.*, p. 148.

69. According to Barthes, not all texts are capable of being 'read' in this way, particularly 'classical' texts. He referred to these classical texts that are open to only a single reading as 'readerly' *(lisible)*, and to 'modern' texts capable of multiple readings as 'writerly' *(scriptible)*.

70. Johnson, B. *The Critical Difference*, Baltimore: John Hopkins University Press, 1980, p. 5.

71. See, for example, Barthes, R. (1973) *The Pleasure of the Text*, New York: Hill & Wang, 1975; and Barthes, R. (1975) *Roland Barthes by Roland Barthes*, London: Macmillan Press, 1995.

72. Barthes, R. (1971) Writers, intellectuals, teachers. In R. Barthes *Image Music Text*, London: Fontana, 1977, p. 201, original emphasis.

73. Payne, M. *Reading Theory*, Oxford: Blackwell, 1993, p. 121, original emphasis.

74. Derrida, *op. cit.*, p. 158.

75. *Ibid.*, p. 9. Derrida often referred to this extended concept as 'arche-writing'.

76. *Ibid.*, p. 157.

77. *Ibid.*, p. lxxvii.

78. Usher and Edwards, *op. cit.*, p. 120.

79. *Ibid.*, p. 124.

80. Some writers see post-structuralism and postmodernism as essentially the

same, so that 'when... philosophers use the word "postmodernism" they mean to refer to a movement that developed in France in the 1960s, more precisely called "poststructuralism", along with subsequent and related developments': Cahoone, *op. cit.*, p. 2.

81. Lyotard, J.-F. (1979) *The Postmodern Condition: A Report on Knowledge,* Manchester: Manchester University Press, 1984.

82. Although Foucault, in the mid-1960s, anticipated a 'post' modern age that would follow his *episteme* of modernism. The modern age saw the birth of 'man' (Foucault's term) as a self-aware being, able to study himself and act reflexively. Thus 'man is an invention of recent date. And one perhaps nearing its end': Foucault, M. (1966) *The Order of Things*, London: Tavistock, 1970, p. 387. Just as the classical age made way for the modern age, so too, Foucault speculated, might the modern age, the age of man, make way for a post modern age in which 'man would be erased, like a face drawn in the sand at the edge of the sea': *Ibid.*, p. 387.

83. Jameson, F. Foreword. In Lyotard, *op. cit.*, 1984, p. vii.

84. Lyotard, J-F. (1982) Answer to the question: what is the postmodern? In J.-F. Lyotard *The Postmodern Explained to Children*, London: Turnaround, 1992, p. 17.

85. Baudrillard, J. (1981) *Simulations*, New York: Semiotext(e), 1983.

86. Lyotard (1982), *op cit.*, p. 8. In other words, what counts as scientific knowledge is determined by 'legislators' such as journal editors.

87. Foucault, M. *Power/Knowledge; Selected Interviews and Other Writings 1972–77*, C. Gordon (ed.) Brighton: Harvester Press, 1980, p. 131.

88. Lyotard (1982), *op. cit.*, pp. 8–9.

89. Bhaskar, R. *The Possibility of Naturalism: A Critique of the Contemporary Human Sciences*, Brighton: Harvester Press, 1979, p. 73.

90. Or what he later referred to as 'critical realism'. Bhaskar, R. (1988) What is critical realism? In R. Bhaskar *Reclaiming Reality*, London: Verso, 1989, p. 190.

91. Bhaskar, R. (1979) Realism in the natural sciences. In R. Bhaskar *Reclaiming Reality*, London: Verso, 1989, p. 23.

92. Bhaskar (1988) *op. cit.*, p. 191. The ongoing debate between the realists and the postmodernists is, of course, far more complex than the simplified account I have given here.

93. Wittgenstein, L. (1921) *Tractatus Logico-philosophicus*, D.F. Pears and B.F. McGuiness (trans.), London: Routledge & Kegan Paul, 1961, 6.35.

94. Bhaskar (1979) *op. cit.*, p. 13.

95. Rorty, *op cit.*, p. 5.

96. *Ibid.* p. 5.

97. Rorty, R. *Objectivity, Relativism, and Truth: Philosophical Papers*, Volume 1, Cambridge, Cambridge University Press, 1991, p. 12.

98. Rorty, R. (1985) Solidarity or objectivity. In *ibid.*, p. 23, original emphasis.

99. Brown, R.H. Reconstructing social theory after the postmodern critique. In H.W. Simons and M. Billig (eds) *After Postmodernism: Reconstructing Ideology Critique*, London: Sage, 1994, p. 27.

100. Smart, *op. cit.*, p. 103.
101. It is worth considering the distinction made by Hans-Georg Gadamer between being *in* authority (that is, having power) and being *an* authority (that is, having knowledge). See Gadamer, H.-G. *The Enigma of Health*, Cambridge: Polity, 1996, pp. 117–24. This issue will be developed further in the next chapter.
102. Usher and Edwards, *op. cit.*, p. 147.
103. That is, postmodernism is arguing against *scientism*, which has been defined as 'the belief that science, especially natural science, is much the most valuable part of human learning – much the most valuable part because it is much the most authoritative, or serious, or beneficial'. Sorell, *op. cit.*, p. 1. However, the philosopher Hilary Putnam claimed that the relativist view was equally scientistic. Thus, 'the scientistic character of logical positivism is quite overt and unashamed; but I think there is a scientism behind relativism. The theory that all there is to "rationality" is what your local culture says it is... is a scientistic theory inspired by anthropology': Putnam, H. *Reason, Truth and History*, Cambridge: Cambridge University Press, 1981, p. 126.
104. Sokal, A. and Bricmont, J. (1997) *Intellectual Impostures*, London: Profile Books, 1998.
105. *Ibid.*, back cover.
106. Henley, J. Euclidean, Spinozist or existentialist? Er, no. It's simply a load of old tosh, *Guardian*, 1 October, 1997, p. 3.
107. Sokal and Bricmont, *op. cit.*, Appendices A–C, pp. 199–258.
108. *Ibid.*, pp. ix–x.
109. *Ibid.*, p. 4.
110. *Ibid.*, p. 11.
111. *Ibid.*, p. 6.
112. *Ibid.*, p. 11.
113. *Ibid.*, p. 173.
114. *Ibid.*, p. 12.
115. *Ibid.*, p. 13.
116. *Ibid.*, review from the *Independent on Sunday*, cited on the front cover of the English language edition of the book.
117. *Ibid.*, p. x.
118. *Ibid.*, p. 49.
119. *Ibid.*, p. 51.
120. *Ibid.*, p. 173.
121. *Ibid.*, p. 51.
122. *Ibid.*, p. 4.
123. *Ibid.*, p. 176.
124. *Ibid.*, p. 176.
125. *Ibid.*, p. 51.
126. *Ibid.*, p. 173.
127. *Ibid.*, p. 193.

CHAPTER THREE

Beyond relativism:
making choices in a decentred universe

*Here they are no longer talking of what is Good & Evil,
or of what is Right or Wrong, & puzzling themselves in Satan's Labyrinth,
But are Conversing with Eternal Realities as they Exist
in the Human Imagination*[1]

TRUTH, POWER AND AUTHORITY

In the previous two chapters, I have tried to show how the history of the development of science is also the history of the development of our concept of truth. In the prescientific age before the sixteenth century, truth was usually defined in Europe according to the grand narrative of religion, and was based on an appeal to faith. So, for example, the Earth was considered to be at the centre of the Universe because this was written in the Bible, and we were expected to accept it as true because we had faith in God, and in the Bible as the word of God.

This established view was first put under pressure by the work of the astronomer Nicolas Copernicus in the mid-sixteenth century with the publication of *De Revolutionibus Orbium*, a theoretical description of a heliocentric (sun-centred) universe. However, it was Galileo who confirmed this theory in the following century with empirical observations, thereby initiating a shift in the world-view to a grand narrative of scientific empiricism, truth being based on an appeal to observation and reason. Thus, the Earth was now considered to be a minor planet revolving around the sun because it was written in the works of scientists and philosophers, and we were expected to accept it as true because we accepted the scientific method as the most effective means of discovering the truth.

This rationalist grand narrative was gradually superseded by a technological one during the nineteenth century, so that truth was established not so much by an appeal to what was rational, but to what was practical; the appeal to reason was therefore replaced by an appeal to utility. Part of the cause of this shift was no doubt the growing complexity of the scientific world-view and the inability to express scientific truths in anything other than a complex mathematical language. Thus, whereas the Newtonian conception of a mechanical universe was readily understood by the layperson, the Einsteinian universe is 'not only stranger than we imagine, but stranger than we *can* imagine';[2] in other words, it is literally inconceivable. Similarly with the products of technology: early machines and gadgets could be readily understood and repaired by almost anyone, whereas in the computer age, most gadgets are 'black boxes' whose internal workings are a mystery to all but a few experts. The truth of a scientific concept is therefore less to do with whether it is rational and understandable than with whether it has practical applications. If subatomic physics can result in nuclear power stations, we accept the theory underpinning it as being true, even though we might have no understanding of that theory.

It is tempting to think of this succession of grand narratives as moving ever closer to a 'true' concept of truth, but as we saw in the previous chapter, this notion has been challenged by the postmodernists, who have expressed an 'attitude of incredulity' towards *all* grand narratives. The successive appeals to faith, reason and utility are equally flawed because they are all essentially appeals to an authority based not on knowledge but on power. From this perspective, the shift from the grand narrative of religion to that of rationality, and then to that of technology, is really a reflection of the shift in the power base from the church, to state-funded science, to industry and big business. And the ultimate breakdown of *all* grand narratives has led finally to a free-for-all in which power is up for grabs by anyone.

So, for example, the shift in grand narratives from religion to rationality is exemplified[3] by Galileo's disagreement with the Church over whether the Earth revolved around the sun or vice versa. This was clearly far more than a dispute about knowledge; it was a struggle to establish the authority by which knowledge could be defined, a power struggle. Similarly, the recent disputes between governments and corporate businesses, such as MacDonalds' cultivation of the Brazilian rainforests and Microsoft's perceived attempts to monopolize the computer industry, can be seen as part of a global shift from the grand narrative of science and the state to that of industry and commerce, or even as a scramble for dominance by the individual little narratives of particular businesses: the 'MacDonaldization' or the 'Disneyfication' of the world. Once again, the issue is less about who knows best, than about who has the greater power, in other words, who has authority.

As Gadamer has pointed out, the term 'authority' has two different but related meanings.[4] He distinguishes between being *authoritarian* (that is, being *in* authority) and being *authoritative* (that is, being *an* authority). Being authoritarian clearly involves *assuming* a position of authority, and in epistemological terms, it is the forcible imposition of knowledge or of a grand narrative onto someone in a less powerful position. In contrast, being authoritative involves *being given* a position of authority, since no one can simply claim to be an authority on a particular issue. This kind of authority is gained by consensus, and has to be granted by a wider community.

So, for example, the government might impose compulsory educational testing for all seven-year-olds, underpinned by the argument that these tests can meaningfully distinguish between good and bad schools. Since the government is *in* authority, it is able and entitled to carry out this action, and, more significantly, to promote its views that the information generated by such tests results in valid knowledge. However, a leading academic might argue that these tests are of no practical use in determining the relative merits of different schools, and should be scrapped. Since this academic is *an* authority, she is equally entitled to promote her view that the tests produce nothing but meaningless statistics. In such a conflict, the outcome (and hence, what is generally perceived as the truth) will largely depend on the relative strengths of the political authority of the government and the epistemological authority of the academic. The government, however, is usually in the stronger position, and often explicitly calls into question the epistemological authority of the academic. Thus, for example, it has been noted how the Conservative government employed the 'discourse of derision' in the 1988 Education Reform Act in order to:

> debunk and displace not only specific words and meanings – progressivism and comprehensivism, for example – but also the speakers of these words, those 'experts', 'specialists' and 'professionals' referred to as the 'educational establishment'.[5]

Authoritarianism, however, often works in far more subtle ways. For example, it might seem that the authority of science is based on epistemological truth (being *an* authority) rather than political truth (being *in* authority). However, as Lyotard pointed out:

> It is recognised that the conditions of truth, in other words the rules of the game of science, are immanent in that game, that they can only be established within the bounds of a debate that is already scientific in nature, and that there is no other proof that the rules are good than the consensus extended to them by the experts.[6]

In other words, what counts as truth in science is not objectively determined, but is established by scientists themselves, and is therefore open to political distortion: 'the game of science is thus put on a par with others'.[7] Those in authority are well aware that science is a game with rules that can be bent to suit their own needs. Therefore, rather than setting itself up in opposition to scientific opinion, as in the above example from education, the government often finds it more expedient to buy off the experts. As Lyotard pointed out:

> the State spends large amounts of money to enable science to pass itself off as an epic: the State's own credibility is based on that epic, which it uses to obtain the public consent its decision makers need.[8]

Thus, 'scientists, technicians, and instruments are purchased not to find truth, but to augment power'.[9] Scientists are therefore often placed in the uncomfortable position of being, at the same time, *in* authority and *an* authority.

This conflict between being in authority and being an authority results in two different ways of looking at truth. On the one hand, truth is defined by those with power, and therefore has a political agenda, leading ultimately to dictatorship.[10] Foucault, for example, argued that truth and power are two sides of the same political coin and cannot be considered separately. Thus, 'we are subjected to the production of truth through power and we cannot exercise power except through the production of truth'.[11] On the other hand, truth is defined by those with knowledge and has an epistemological agenda. Arguably, this latter conception of truth is essential for the survival of a democratic system of government, in which the dissemination of truth must be divorced from political power.[12] The implications of 'truth' being disseminated by those with political power can be seen, for example, in the recent controversy over information about the transmission of bovine spongiform encephalopathy (BSE) to humans, in which the Ministry of Agriculture clearly had a political agenda to protect British farming interests as well as an epistemological agenda to disseminate the truth about BSE, resulting in a series of half-truths about the possible consequences of eating beef.[13]

From the postmodern perspective, if we wish to move away from power and towards knowledge as the defining characteristic of truth, we must reject those who are *in* authority in favour of those who are *an* authority, and that entails rejecting grand narratives *(grands récits)* in favour of what Lyotard called 'little narratives' *(petits récits)*. For Lyotard, a grand narrative claims to tell (and, therefore, to authorize) *the* story of which little narratives form disjointed and incomplete parts; it is thus 'the story that can reveal the meaning of all stories... so as to reveal the singular truth inherent in all of them'.[14] So, for example, the grand narrative of science is the (authoritarian) epistemological framework that legitimates the various little narratives of methodologies, research findings and so on.

For Lyotard, however, the grand narratives of the Enlightenment project have broken down, his symbol for the failure of modernism being, as we saw in the previous chapter, Auschwitz. Thus, 'I have used the name "Auschwitz" to signify just how impoverished recent Western history seems from the point of view of the "modern" project of the emancipation of humanity.'[15] Grand narratives, and in particular the grand narrative of emancipation through scientific rationality, have failed us: rather than emancipation, they have exerted ever greater control (Lyotard provides the example of totalitarian communist states); rather than a better life, they have resulted in weapons of mass destruction (the Holocaust, Hiroshima); rather than equality, they have resulted in 'the growing gap between the wealth of the North and the impoverished South, unemployment and the "new poor"'.[16.]

But in rejecting grand narratives as providing solutions to the problems faced by humanity, all we are left with is a succession of 'little narratives', each of which follows on from the others, such that:

> The serial disposition of little narratives (one simply comes after another, and so on in non-finite series) means that no one narrative can become the master [grand] narrative organizing the field of language-elements.[17]

For Lyotard, these little narratives roughly corresponded to what Wittgenstein called 'language games',[18] by which he meant the multiplicity of uses to which language is put, and the different rules that structure those uses, 'in exactly the same way as a game of chess is defined by a set of rules determining the properties of each of the pieces'.[19] As Lyotard pointed out, however, there are a number of observations to be made about language games. First, the rules of each game are not externally set, but are agreed upon by the players. Second, if there are no rules, there is no game. And third, every utterance should be thought of as a 'move' in a game.[20] It is therefore impossible to step outside language games in order to judge them from an objective perspective, so that none is entitled to make a claim of superiority over any other. In rejecting grand narratives in favour of little narratives, we also reject authoritarian knowledge in favour of authoritative knowledge.

THE LIBERAL IRONIST

The postmodernists, then, reject those who are *in* authority in favour of those who are *an* authority as establishing the rules and criteria for the generation and dissemination of knowledge. As we have seen, however, this implies an epistemological shift from a single grand narrative to a series of little narratives, none of which can claim superiority over any other. However, there is a growing movement (or, more accurately, a fairly loose configuration of writers and writings), including Stuart Hall's 'Marxism without guarantees'[21] and Assiter's 'modernist feminism',[22] as well as literary theorists and sociologists, that is unhappy with some of the implications of this shift towards little narratives.

On the one hand, it is objected, postmodernists are claiming that all little narratives have an equal claim to the truth, resulting in a 'moral quietism'[23] in which a commitment to any cause is viewed as naïve. On the other hand, it is pointed out that, despite its relativist rhetoric that all little narratives are equal, the postmodern narrative considers itself to be superior to all others. Thus, 'Texts may be everything, but relativists' texts, it seems, occupy a privileged position',[24] a position that is upheld by a variety of subtle means such as the selective use of inverted commas 'to maintain distinctions between that which they wish to analyse as constructed and that which they hold to be real'.[25]

The literary critic and Marxist Terry Eagleton developed this point further, arguing that the postmodernist project of deconstructing discourses of power is itself 'a power-game, a mirror-image of orthodox academic competition'.[26] This view was reinforced by the feminist Rosalind Gill, for whom 'discursive analyses... are not – and cannot be – value-free',[27] and who went on to point out that 'paradoxically, epistemological sceptics seem to have reinstated, rather than challenged, the notion of value-freedom in research'.[28]

These critics appear to be confusing the postmodern stance of epistemic relativism, the view that each little narrative has an equal claim to knowledge, with that of judgemental relativism, the view that it is therefore not possible to judge between little narratives. Also, as we have seen, this misrepresentation has left postmodernism open to charges not only of moral quietism, but also of hypocrisy in placing its own little narrative above those of its competitors.

However, we saw in the previous chapter that it *is* logically possible for postmodernists to make judgements between competing little narratives; indeed, it is essential that they do so, since even the most ardent epistemic relativist would presumably wish to make ethical choices and even epistemological ones. After all, as Gill suggested, above, all postmodernists have chosen the discourse of postmodernism over competing discourses.

In fact, Lyotard devoted an entire book to the subject of how it is possible to judge between competing positions, or what he referred to as 'phrases'.[29] The difficulty, as he saw it, was that the construction of phrases depends on sets of rules, called phrase regimens,[30] there being 'a number of regimens: reasoning, knowing, describing, recounting, questioning, showing, ordering, and so on'.[31] When there is a dispute between two phrases from the same regimen (what Lyotard called a litigation), it can be settled in a more or less rational fashion by a neutral judge applying the rules of that particular regimen. However, a problem arises when phrases from different regimens come into conflict, for example, those of an employee who feels that she has been exploited, and of her employer who claims to have been only following the law. The problem is that to judge the dispute from the phrase regimen of either party is to do an injustice to the other, whereas to judge from a third regimen, as though it had some kind of authority over the other two, is to do them both an injustice.

Such a dispute is referred to, in Lyotard's terminology, as a *differend*, which he defined as 'a case of conflict, between (at least two) parties, that cannot be equitably resolved for lack of a rule applicable to both arguments'.[32] Thus:

> applying a single rule of judgement to both in order to settle their differend as though it were merely a litigation [that is, as though the rule applied equally to both of them] would wrong (at least) one of them (and both of them if neither side admits this rule)... A wrong results from the fact that the rules of the genre of discourse by which one judges are not those of the judged genre or genres of discourse.[33]

In the case of the above example, the employee is citing a moral wrong and deploying an ethical phrase regimen, whereas the employer is denying a legal wrong and deploying a normative phrase regimen. If the dispute is settled in a court of law using the regimen of the employer, the 'plaintiff is deprived of means of arguing, and so becomes a victim'.[34]

So what is to be done? As Lyotard put it:

> Given 1) the impossibility of avoiding conflicts (the impossibility of indifference) and 2) the absence of a universal genre of discourse to regulate them (or, if you prefer, the inevitable partiality of the judge): to find, if not what can legitimate judgement, then at least how to save the honor of thinking.[35]

The problem, then, lies in 'detecting differends and in finding the (impossible) idiom for phrasing them. This is what a philosopher does'.[36] The reason that the philosopher is able to do this (seemingly) impossible task is because her own phrase regimen, her own language game, is different from most others; it is, in Lyotard's words, a 'metalanguage'. But we must be careful here: we have already seen that Lyotard has expressed incredulity towards meta*narratives*, so how does the philosopher's meta*language* differ? As Lyotard pointed out, the difference hinges on the multiple usage of the prefix 'meta' to mean (among other things) 'beyond' and also 'about'. Thus, Lyotard is not using the term 'metalanguage' in what he calls 'the logician's sense'[37] of meaning a language that stands above or beyond ordinary languages, but rather in 'the linguist's sense' of a language that describes and remarks upon other languages; a language *about* language. He is thus using the term 'metalanguage' in the same way that philosophers use the term 'metaethics', that is, not as some form of superior ethical system that can make judgements about other 'lesser' systems, but as 'the second-order activity of investigating the concepts and methods of ethics'.[38]

However, while this definition of a metalanguage as a 'second-order activity' of investigating the concepts and methods of language saves the philosopher's phrase regimen from incredulity, it also means that the philosopher is unable to judge rationally between other competing regimens, and 'in this very way, it denies itself the possibility of settling, on the basis of its own rules, the differends it examines'.[39] All the philosopher can do, then, is to 'bear witness to the differend',[40] to reveal the incommensurability of the two phrase regimens, and to attempt to ensure a fair hearing for both sides. This is not to deny the possibility of a judgement: a decision can still be made, but not on a rational basis, since there is no common ground between the two sides. The decision must therefore be made from the neutral (but not superior) phrase regimen of 'the judgement, the most enigmatic of phrases, *the one which follows no rules*'.[41] Elsewhere, Lyotard expanded on this notion of judgement without rules, and:

> the thinker I am closest to in this regard is Aristotle, insofar as he recognizes... that a judge worthy of the name has no true model to guide his judgements, and that the true nature of the judge is to pronounce judgements, and therefore prescriptions, just so, without criteria. This is, after all, what Aristotle calls prudence. It consists in dispersing justice without models.[42]

Judgements, then, can be made, but they are enigmatic; they follow no rules, for there *are* no rules that would do equal justice to both sides. For this reason, 'the law should always be respected with humor because it cannot be completely respected, except at the price of giving credence to the idea that it is the very mode of linking heterogeneities together [that is, a metanarrative], that it has the necessity of total Being'.[43]

Lyotard is thus not claiming, as some of the critics cited earlier would claim, that the little narrative or discourse of postmodern philosophy has placed itself in a privileged position in relation to other discourses. The 'metalanguage' of the postmodern philosopher is not, as we have seen, an overarching higher-order language *of* language, but a second-order language *about* language. Neither, however, does it fall into the trap of relativism, since, as one writer has pointed out, 'there is a distinction between indeterminate judgement and a relativist refusal to judge, a pluralist insistence that all judgements are equally valid'.[44] The postmodern philosopher is able to make judgements between different phrase regimens precisely because she recognizes that all such judgements are essentially (to use Lyotard's term) enigmatic: they follow no rules. It is in this sense that Lyotard claimed (see above) that the law should be respected with humour; it should be regarded playfully rather than seriously, since all its judgements are, in a way, arbitrary. The authority (authoritativeness) that allows the postmodernist philosopher to judge is therefore her recognition that she has no authority (authoritarianism).

But if ethical and epistemological judgements are possible in a postmodern world, then so is commitment, and 'there is no contradiction... between being a relativist and being a fully paid-up member of a particular culture with commitments and a commonsense notion of reality'.[45] Thus, it is possible, while holding fast to many of the tenets of postmodernism, to develop a 'passionately interested inquiry'[46] or 'politically informed relativism'.[47]

One writer who has done more than most to pave the way for a return to political commitment as a *development* of postmodernism rather than a *reaction* to it, is the American philosopher Richard Rorty. Rorty attempted to reconcile the contingency of language evident in the work of Lyotard and Derrida with the 'passionately interested enquiry' of the new feminists. For Rorty, it is not the world that is true or false – that is a quite meaningless concept – but our descriptions of it. And those descriptions can only be made within a language, which is, of course, a human creation. Thus, although the world might exist independently of people, truth cannot. Therefore:

To say that truth is not out there is simply to say that where there are no sentences there is no truth, that sentences are elements of human languages, and that human languages are human creations.[48]

Truth is therefore contingent on the human creation of language, and 'human beings make truths by making languages in which to phrase sentences'.[49] However, Rorty was careful not to fall into the self-referential inconsistency of relativism and its ultimate recourse to moral quietism. Thus, he continued by emphasizing that:

To say that we should drop the idea of truth as out there waiting to be discovered is not to say that we have discovered that, out there, there is no truth.[50]

In fact, Rorty had little interest in whether there was a truth 'out there', since in practical terms it made little difference. Instead, he was concerned with how individuals lived and worked with their own conceptions of truth, constructed through what he called their 'final vocabularies'. These final vocabularies are 'the words in which we tell... the story of our lives',[51] and consist of the vocabulary that makes up our view of the world, or *Weltanschauung*. Some of these words, such as 'good', 'right' and 'beautiful', are value laden, whereas others are terms that those value words describe, such as 'the Church', 'England' and 'education'. Our final vocabularies, then, are the words we use to describe who we are and what we believe.

We have already seen that, for Rorty, truth resides in language, more specifically in sentences. Thus, when I say, 'Education is good', I am expressing what for me is a truth (unless, of course, I am deliberately lying). However, the status of this truth can be understood in a number of ways. It can be understood in the modernist sense as a universal truth, as true for all time in all situations and for all people, that is, as part of some grand narrative such as that of the Enlightenment project. Conversely, it can be seen from a postmodernist perspective as a little narrative, as an expression of belief that has no more or less truth-value than any other little narrative. However, Rorty outlined a third position, which occupies the middle ground between the two extremes. He claimed that the statement 'Education is good' could also be uttered 'ironically', that is, with the recognition that the statement is contingent, but also with a commitment to its claim to be the 'best' description of the world, whatever the term 'best' might mean to the individual.

For Rorty, an ironist is someone who fulfils three conditions. First, she has radical doubts about her own final vocabulary because she has been impressed by the final vocabularies of others with whom she has come into contact, either in person or through their writing. Second, she realizes that those doubts cannot be resolved by arguments phrased in her own final vocabulary; that is, her argument that education is good can never fully triumph over the argument, for example, that education is a restrictive social force. Third, she does not believe *her* final vocabulary to be closer to reality than any other; that is, there are no higher powers underwriting certain final vocabularies.[52] The ironist, then, has made a choice, but cannot logically defend her choice against the choices made by others. Thus, the ironist, unlike the judgemental relativist, is not in a state of nihilistic despair. She still has a project to which she can commit herself, although she cannot validate her project by an appeal to some external grand narrative. She simply *believes* her project to be the best, at the same time knowing that there is no epistemological substance to her belief.

Rorty is quite explicit about his own project, his own choice of final vocabulary. He describes himself as a liberal, borrowing the definition from Judith Shklar, 'who says that liberals are the people who think that cruelty is the worst thing we do'.[53] However, Rorty is, of course, also an ironist, someone who acknowledges that his chosen final vocabulary is no more defensible than that of anyone else. Thus, 'for liberal ironists, there is no answer to the question "Why not be cruel?" – no noncircular theoretical backup for the belief that cruelty is horrible'.[54]

This combination of modernist liberalism and postmodernist irony is a curious mix, particularly since we saw in the previous chapter that postmodernism is not so much a successor to modernism as a critique of it. Rorty was quick to acknowledge that liberalism and ironism are strange bedfellows, citing as the main influences on his position that staunch defender of modernism against the postmodern menace, Jürgen Habermas, and the post-structuralist and critic of modernism, Michel Foucault. Thus, 'Michel Foucault is an ironist who is unwilling to be a liberal, whereas Jürgen Habermas is a liberal who is unwilling to be an ironist'.[55]

This mix of ironism and liberalism introduces a major dilemma for the liberal ironist when she comes to disseminate her views to others, since the ironist position has the interesting effect of dissociating truth from knowledge. My claim that education is good cannot be backed up by an argument based on knowledge, since my knowledge is shaped by the final vocabulary that I have chosen to express my claim, which might be different from your final vocabulary. Yet I wish to assert the truth of my statement, and I wish for you, too, to accept it as true. Because we do not share a common final vocabulary, however, I cannot persuade you by rational argument, nor by recourse to research-based knowledge; instead, I must somehow *impose* my truth on you. As a liberal, however, I clearly cannot impose my truth by force, since I also oppose cruelty. The solution for Rorty:

> is to redescribe lots and lots of things in new ways, until you have created a pattern of linguistic behavior which will tempt the rising generation to adopt it, thereby causing them to look for appropriate new forms of nonlinguistic behavior... It says things like 'try thinking of it this way' – or more specifically, 'try to ignore the apparently futile traditional questions by substituting the following new and possibly interesting questions.'[56]

Thus, the aim of the liberal ironist is not the pursuit of rational or empirical knowledge, since rational arguments fall apart once they leave the final vocabularies in which they were formulated. Her aim is instead to redescribe the world in terms of her own particular final vocabulary in the hope that others might adopt it as their own. She would not, then, say, 'YOU must do it this way because research says this way is best', but 'Try it this way because you might find that it will work better.' It is therefore a political rather than an epistemological project, although, being liberal, it is concerned with the politics of consensus rather than of power.

RESEARCH AND THE IRONIST

In the course of the three chapters that make up Part I of this book, I have outlined three positions on knowledge and truth. The first was the modernist view of an absolute truth, of an objective knowledge that exists independently of the knower, and of the methods of empirical scientific research as the best, or even the only, way of gaining access to that knowledge. The second was the 'classic' or generally held postmodernist view that there are no grand narratives to which we can appeal, that all knowledge claims are equally valid, and hence that there is no such thing as absolute truth. Third came Rorty's liberal ironist position, in which grand narratives are looked upon with incredulity, but in which certain little narratives are epistemologically superior to others because they are aware of their own contingency. I will now consider some of the implications for the researcher (in particular, the nurse researcher) of each of these positions.

The modernist researcher

The fundamental concern of modernist scientific research, which can be seen from most definitions, is with producing generalizable knowledge. The aim of research is to be able to make general statements that apply beyond the subjects on whom the research is being carried out, and the scientific method is employed to ensure that the research findings are suitably decontextualized and depersonalized. The researcher takes great care to ensure that the findings of the research are disassociated from the place and the situation in which they were generated, from the subjects from whom they were generated, and from the researcher who generated them (that is, from herself). All influences of people, places and situations are therefore written out of the research, which is presented as being neutral and objective. The application of method, then, is seen as the guarantee of generalizability and objectivity: if the rules of the scientific method are rigidly followed, whatever findings emerge must be valid not only for the subjects from whom they were generated, but also for a wider population. Thus, the little narratives of particular research methods are underwritten by the metanarrative of scientific Method.[57]

From the modernist perspective, then, knowledge cannot be separated from research, and science is seen as a universal language in which judgements about truths within any particular discipline can be made, solely by an appeal to Method. As Phillips pointed out, 'we do not consult what a proposition proposes, we consult the rules [of scientific Method] used to decide if what the proposition proposes is warranted'.[58] This rather extreme interpretation of the technical rationality paradigm has found its strongest voice in the medical and paramedical professions, where it is proposed that clinical decisions should be based on an evaluation of research findings rather than on an appeal to the authority of expert practitioners. Thus:

> The new paradigm [of evidence-based medicine] puts a much lower value on authority. The underlying belief is that physicians can gain the skills to make independent assessments of [research] evidence and thus evaluate the credibility of opinions being offered by experts.[59]

Valuing the findings of research above expert opinion might, on the face of it, appear to be a laudable intention, but taken to its logical conclusion, it suggests that clinical decisions are ultimately decisions about the way in which research is conducted, rather than about medicine. As Phillips suggested (see above), the practitioner is not assessing the clinical worth of the findings, but is making a judgement about whether the rules of research have been properly adhered to in arriving at the findings.

This approach to practice has a number of important consequences. It implies that, in judging the truth of the findings of medical research, all that is really needed is an understanding of research methods. This, in turn, suggests that a sociologist or a psychologist could make a judgement about the findings of a piece of medical research merely by critiquing the methods employed to arrive at those findings, without any knowledge of medical theory or practice.[60] The educationalist Lawrence Stenhouse was very critical of this position, pointing out that:

> without understanding why one course of action is better than another, we could prove by statistical treatment that it is. The vision is an enticing one: it suggests that we may make wise judgements without understanding what we are doing.[61]

The danger for Stenhouse was that judgements made from the perspective of the metanarrative of science, judgements made solely on the criteria of 'good science', would override the professional or technical judgements made from the perspective of the little narrative of professional practice by practitioners themselves.

We can see, then, that Method is the defining attribute of scientific research, that the findings of research are guaranteed their validity through strict adherence to Method, and as Phillips pointed out, our judgement of the validity of research findings is essentially a judgement about the way in which the research was conducted. Method takes on an authoritarian function; as Barthes observed, 'Method becomes a Law',[62] a metanarrative. For the modernists, research has an 'end' in both meanings of the word: it has the clear goal (end-point) of the discovery of knowledge, and thus the potential for termination (ending) with either the perfection of Method or the achievement of the goal of knowing all that there is to know, or at least, all that is worth knowing.[63]

The 'classical' postmodern researcher

In contrast to this modernist perspective lies the 'classical' or popularly held postmodern view that we live in a decentred universe without absolute truths. Postmodernists claim that there are no metanarratives or overarching explanations of how the world works, but only a succession of little narratives, or partial and contingent accounts,

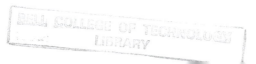

including the little narrative of science. Scientific research, then, does not provide us with access to the truth, because there is no single truth; instead, it offers *one* method for constructing knowledge[64] that is no more privileged than any other method. Thus:

> great scientists invent descriptions of the world which are useful for purposes of predicting and controlling what happens, just as poets and political thinkers invent other descriptions of it for other purposes. But there is no sense in which *any* of these descriptions is an accurate representation of the way the world is in itself.[65]

This view of science as a little narrative should not necessarily cause us to reject the claim of evidence-based practice, that, for example, the knowledge base of nursing should be founded on scientific research. However, such a claim would not have a privileged position over claims from nurses themselves that the knowledge base should be founded on experience, or from doctors that it should be founded on medicine. Thus:

> instead of hovering above, legitimation descends to the level of practice and becomes immanent in it. There are no special tribunals set apart from the sites where inquiry is practised. Rather, practitioners assume responsibility for legitimizing their own practice.[66]

As we have seen, postmodernists argue that knowledge cannot be separated from power, since power usually includes the authority to define what counts as knowledge: the person who is *in* authority is often in a position to decide who is *an* authority. Thus, the claim for science would be one little narrative among many, and it would have to be made *not*, as is currently the case, from an authoritarian position, but from an authoritative one. By dissociating power from truth by the rejection of metanarratives, the postmodernist hopes to disperse the authority of a discipline among all of its participants.

The narrative of science would therefore not be in a position to impose itself as *the* method of verifying truth claims in nursing, but would, according to Rorty, have to redescribe the world in its own terms in the hope that nurses and others with an interest in the discipline would adopt its narrative in their own final vocabularies.[67] The problem, of course, is that in adopting an attitude of incredulity towards *all* narratives, we have no way of choosing between them. If science does not provide us with the truth, neither do any of the alternatives to science. In throwing out the bathwater of the authoritarian scientific Method, we are forced also into throwing out the baby of the possibility of *any* method offering a more authoritative account of truth than any other.

The postmodern ironist researcher

This brings us to the third position, which argues against the total relativism of the 'classical' postmodernist position in favour of a partial 'ironic' relativism. This ironist position accepts epistemic relativism, the view that knowledge is socially constructed and is, as such, contingent on the knower, but rejects judgemental relativism, the argument that we cannot, or may not, judge between different truth claims. Thus, whereas classical postmodernists are incredulous towards the methods of science, but have nothing to replace them with, postmodern ironists reject the authoritarian *Method* of science in favour of certain authoritative *methods* (in a very loose sense of the term).[68] Of course, from a total relativist position, we are unable to make *any* sort of informed judgement between methods. However, you might recall Lyotard's argument that the postmodern philosopher is able to make 'enigmatic' judgements, judgements without rules based on a metalanguage that can represent all sides in a dispute; in Rorty's terminology, the postmodernist philosopher judges ironically.

Thus, just as the postmodern ironist researcher rejects the scientific method as a metanarrative that claims to offer a justification for all other methods, while requiring no justification for itself, so she advocates for ironist research methods that are formulated in the full understanding that there is no logical basis for them; they are simply thought to be the best possible methods in the circumstances, and no attempt is made to impose them forcibly on anyone else. The ironist simply tries to describe her position in the most attractive way possible so that the listener might recognize it as being a better description of the world than that which she currently holds.

This notion of accepting the (epistemological) authority of ironist methods over the (methodological) authority of scientific Method might appear to be a dangerous move for the nurse researcher. After all, scientific research is built on a firm empirical foundation and is open to scrutiny, unlike ironist methods, which acknowledge their contingency and fallibility. An ironist method, then, is only accepted by consensus, by those people who share its little narrative, and rational argument has little effect in changing the opinions of others, since they play different language games. The power of language is not in its appeal to logic, but in its ability to describe the world in terms that others might find attractive. However, this is the point at which we begin to run up against self-referential arguments. The ironist cannot (indeed, will not) offer a rational argument for her position – she merely states it – and there is no logical reason why anyone should adopt it over 'rational' modernist science. Then again, from the ironist perspective, there is no reason why anyone should not: they are simply two statements, two 'phrase regimes' (to use Lyotard's terminology), which speak different languages. Just as a German speaker has no way of communicating to a French speaker why German is a superior language to French (and vice versa), so the ironist researcher has no way of communicating to the modernist researcher why ironic research is superior to traditional research.

It would appear, then, that the rather complex philosophical arguments presented in Part I of this book have resulted in some fairly simple conclusions.[69] First, it is claimed, the discourse of science is a little narrative that believes itself to be a grand narrative, and which acts accordingly. Its status as the driving force of modernism is therefore achieved by its ability to shout louder than other competing little narratives. Second, the 'classical' or commonly understood version of postmodernism argues that all little narratives have equal claims to the truth, and there is thus no way of judging between them. In the realm of epistemology, then, anything goes. Third, postmodern ironists claim that certain little narratives are superior precisely because they recognize that they are little narratives. Thus, the little narratives of ironist research are superior to the little narrative of the Enlightenment project because the latter does not accept that it is a little narrative, but rather asserts that it can (potentially) provide the answers to all the problems of the world. It is therefore the insight and self-awareness of the ironist researcher, her ability to know the limits of her knowledge and power, which results in her superior epistemological position.

CONCLUSION

In Part I of this book, I have briefly surveyed the development of empiricism as the driving force of the Enlightenment project, from its roots in the seventeenth century science of Bacon and Galileo, through the empiricist philosophy of Hume and Locke and the pragmatism of James and Pierce, to the logical positivists of the twentieth century. I also explored the growing tide of objections to scientific empiricism, from the post-positivist critique of the *means* of empirical science to the postmodernist critique of its *ends* and of its privileged position as the only method of establishing valid knowledge. I concluded by discussing Rorty's attempt to reconcile the contingency of postmodernism with the liberal commitment of the

Enlightenment project, and very briefly sketched out the possibility of a postmodern ironist approach to research.

This challenge to the authority (in both meanings of the word) of empirical scientific research has enormous implications for all research-based disciplines, and some, such as anthropology, are already beginning to address the issues.[70] Unfortunately, many others, including nursing, continue to see academic credibility in terms of a close adherence to the methods of science, and are even suspicious of some of the more esoteric modernist methodologies. It is easy to predict, then, what many leading nurse theorists and academics would make of the application of postmodern ironism to nursing: that nurses should base their practice around a variety of 'ironist' research methods rather than on the findings of scientific research; on appeals to intuition and the emotions rather than on appeals to reason. However, as we have seen in the preceding chapters, power and knowledge have become closely entwined, and those with the power to dismiss new ideas do not always possess the knowledge with which to make those judgements; in the terminology of this book, they are often *in* authority without necessarily being *an* authority. Furthermore, their positions of power within the grand narrative of nursing are often dependent on upholding the values of that grand narrative. A leading academic with a dozen research papers to her name and a six-figure research grant is hardly likely to promote the idea that modernist research might not, after all, be the most effective method of generating knowledge and validating truth.

There are, however, a growing number of writers who are arguing for a new authority both in and on nursing, indeed for a new epistemology. Part I of this book has suggested that a different approach to generating and validating knowledge is not only possible, but is also already beginning to be felt in the disciplines of both science and philosophy, although different writers have expressed this new epistemology in different ways and with different degrees of success. In Part II, I will go on to explore some of the many and varied ways in which nurse academics are beginning to challenge the modernist research agenda, illustrating these new perspectives with published examples from journal papers.

NOTES

1. Blake, W. *The Last Judgement*, 1818.
2. Attributed to Carl Sagan.

3. I have deliberately used the word 'exemplified' rather than 'initiated' to conform to Michel Foucault's notion of *epistemes*. As we saw in Chapter 1, Foucault identified a number of historical periods, starting with the Renaissance, which are underpinned and driven by intellectual 'archives' of taken-for-granted assumptions. These infra-structural archives or *epistemes* exist prior to the social, artistic and scientific achievements of any particular age; thus, the great men and women of the age do not determine the *episteme*, but are determined by it. From Foucault's perspective, the *episteme* of the 'Classical Age' (which followed that of the Renaissance) *enabled* Galileo to challenge the authority of the Church rather than Galileo's challenge ushering in a new scientific age: Foucault, M. (1966) *The Order of Things: An Archaeology of the Human Sciences*, London: Tavistock, 1970.

4. Gadamer, H.-G. *The Enigma of Health*, Cambridge: Polity, 1996, pp. 117–24.

5. Ball, S. *Politics and Policy Making in Education: Explorations in Policy Sociology*, London: Routledge, 1990, p. 18.

6. Lyotard, J.-F. (1979) *The Postmodern Condition: A Report on Knowledge*, Manchester: Manchester University Press, 1984, p. 29.

7. *Ibid.*, p. 40.

8. *Ibid.*, pp. 27–8.

9. *Ibid.*, p. 46.

10. This point was made very graphically by George Orwell in his novel *1984*, in which he imagined a dictatorial 'Ministry of Truth' which maintained its power by disseminating lies and rewriting history. Thus, power was employed to shape and define what counted as truth.

11. Foucault, M. *Power/Knowledge: Selected Interviews and Other Writings 1972–1977*, C. Gordon (trans. and ed.), Brighton: Harvester Press, 1986, p. 93.

12. From Foucault's perspective, however, knowledge can *never* be divorced from power. Power relationships are inherent in all social interactions: 'it [power] is produced from one moment to the next, at every point, or rather in every relation from one point to another. Power is everywhere... because it comes from everywhere.' Foucault, M. *The History of Sexuality*, Volume 1: *An Introduction*, London: Allen Lane, 1979, p. 95.

13. Even as I write, the same scenario is being repeated over the issue of genetically modified food.

14. Readings, B. *Introducing Lyotard*, London: Routledge, 1991, p. 63.

15. Lyotard, J.-F. (1985) Note on the meaning of 'post-'. In J.-F. Lyotard *The Postmodern Explained to Children*, London: Turnaround, 1992, p. 91.

16. Lyotard, J.-F. (1985) Ticket for a new stage. In J.-F. Lyotard *The Postmodern Explained to Children*, London: Turnaround, 1992, p. 98.

17. Readings, *op. cit.*, p. 68.

18. Wittgenstein, L. *Philosophical Investigations*, Oxford: Basil Blackwell, 1953.

19. Lyotard, J.-F. (1979) *op. cit.*, p. 10.

20. *Ibid.*, p. 10.

21. Hall, S. The toad in the garden: Thatcherism among the theorists. In C. Nelson and L. Grossberg (eds), *Marxism and the Interpretation of Culture*, London: Macmillan, 1988.

22. Assiter, A. *Enlightened Women: Modernist Feminism in a Postmodern Age*, London: Routledge, 1996.

23. Gill, R. Relativism, reflexivity and politics: interrogating discourse analysis from a feminist perspective. In S. Wilkinson and C. Kitzinger, *Feminism and Discourse: Psychological Perspectives*, London: Sage, 1995, pp. 165–86.

24. *Ibid.*, p. 174.

25. *Ibid.*, p. 171.

26. Eagleton, T. *Literary Theory: An Introduction*, Oxford: Blackwell, 1983, p. 147.

27. Gill, *op. cit.*, p. 175.

28. *Ibid.*, p. 175.

29. Lyotard, J.-F. (1983) *The Differend: Phrases in Dispute*, G. Van Den Abbeele (trans.), Minneapolis: University of Minnesota Press, 1988.

30. Phrase regimens are similar to Kuhn's notion of a paradigm, and to what Wittgenstein called 'language games'.

31. *Ibid.*, p. xii.

32. *Ibid.*, p. xi.

33. *Ibid.*, p. xi.

34. *Ibid.*, p. 30.

35. *Ibid.*, p. xii.

36. As opposed to an intellectual, who is 'someone who helps forget differends, by advocating a different genre... for the sake of political hegemony': *Ibid.*, p. 142.

37. *Ibid.*, p. xiv.

38. Blackburn, S. *The Oxford Dictionary of Philosophy*, Oxford: Oxford University Press, 1994, p. 239.

39. Lyotard, *op. cit.*, p. xiv.

40. *Ibid.*, p. 13.

41. *Ibid.*, p. 149, emphasis added.

42. Lyotard, J.-F. and Thébaud, J.-L. (1985) *Just Gaming*, Minneapolis: University of Minnesota Press, 1979, pp. 25–6.

43. *Ibid.*, p. 144.

44. Readings, *op. cit.* p. 125.

45. Gill, *op cit.*, p. 174.

46. *Ibid.*, p. 175.

47. *Ibid.*, p. 178.

48. Rorty, R. *Contingency, Irony, and Solidarity*, Cambridge: Cambridge University Press, 1989, p. 5.

49. *Ibid.*, p. 9.

50. *Ibid.*, p. 8.

51. *Ibid.*, p. 73. There are clear parallels between Rorty's final vocabularies, Lyotard's phrase regimes, and Wittgenstein's language games.

52. Here, we can see close similarities between Rorty's ironist and Lyotard's postmodern philosopher with her 'enigmatic' judgements.
53. *Ibid.*, p. xv.
54. *Ibid.*, p. xv.
55. *Ibid.*, p. 61.
56. *Ibid.*, p. 9.
57. The use of a capital 'M' for Method follows from the writing of Barthes, and is employed here to distinguish the metanarrative of Method (the rules of science) from the little narratives of individual methods (the application of those rules). Barthes, R. (1971) Writers, intellectuals, teachers. In R. Barthes *Image Music Text*, London: Fontana, 1977, pp. 200–2.
58. Phillips, D.L. *Abandoning Method*, London: Jossey-Bass, 1973, p. 82.
59. Evidence-Based Medicine Working Group. Evidence-based medicine: a new approach to teaching the practice of medicine, *Journal of the American Medical Association*, 1992, **268**, 17, 2421.
60. Its corollary is, of course, that a medical practitioner with no experience of doing research can nevertheless be trained to make judgements about the practice of research, a practice in which she has never participated.
61. Stenhouse, L. Case study and case records: towards a contemporary history of education, *British Educational Research Journal*, 1978, **4**, 2, 21–39.
62. Barthes, *op. cit.*, p. 201.
63. This might seem a very far-fetched goal, but at least one scientist believes that all of the major scientific discoveries are now behind us. Thus, 'there are many tremendously important and exciting things left for scientists to do... But if you want to discover something as monumental as natural selection or general relativity or the big bang theory, if you want to top Darwin or Einstein, your chances are slim to none': Horgan, J. *The End of Science: Facing the Limits of Knowledge in the Twilight of the Scientific Age*, London: Abacus, 1996, p. 271.
64. For postmodernists, knowledge is *constructed* through the use of language rather than *discovered*. It is therefore 'inside us', rather than 'out there' in the world.
65. Rorty, *op. cit.*, p. 4.
66. Fraser, N. and Nicholson, L. Social criticism without philosophy: an encounter between feminism and postmodernism. In A. Ross (ed.) *Universal Abandon? The Politics of Postmodernism*, Edinburgh: Edinburgh University Press, 1988.
67. Rorty, *op. cit.*
68. Of course, once we cut methods free of the tyranny of Method, they can take on a far broader and more imaginative range of approaches to data collection than the rather narrow constraints of the methods of science. A range of possible ironist research methods will be discussed in Part II.
69. The exasperated reader, having got this far, might be wondering at this point why I did not simply spell out the conclusions in the first place without subjecting her to some rather gruelling philosophy. However, that

would be rather like a (modernist) researcher simply stating the recom-
mendations of her study without bothering to write up the method or the
findings, or a mathematician offering the final term in the solution to a
complex problem without bothering with the full mathematical proof. The
whole point of the exercise, from the ironist's perspective, is that she must
convince the reader by persuasion that her story is superior to all other
stories (even though, as we have seen, she cannot rationally justify why it
is superior).

70. See, for example, Denzin, N.K. *Interpretive Ethnography*, London: Sage,
1997; Ellis C. and Bochner A.P. *Composing Ethnography*, Walnut Creek:
AltaMira, 1996; Alasuutari, P. *Researching Culture*, London: Sage, 1995.

PART II

POSTMODERN PERSPECTIVES ON NURSING RESEARCH

*I must Create a System or be enslav'd by another Man's.
I will not Reason and Compare: my business is to Create.*[1]

In Part I of this book, I questioned not only modernism, underpinned by the metanarrative of empirical science, but also its antithesis, the commonly held 'anything goes' version of postmodernism. It is rather ironic that this *laissez-faire* 'anything goes' ethos stems from a profound scepticism, Lyotard's 'incredulity towards metanarratives',[2] and in particular, towards the 'tyranny of Method' that has granted scientific research its epistemological supremacy during the past two hundred years. But of course, this commonly held formulation of postmodernism, like Descartes' 'method of doubt' from three and a half centuries before it, rejected not just the metanarrative of science, but *all* metanarratives, including Marxism, feminism, Christianity and so on. However, the postmodernists, unlike Descartes, did not have God to fall back on.[3] The problem for postmodernism, then, is that if anything goes, how are we to choose between competing little narratives?

I have argued that this commonly held relativist view is a misconception of postmodernism, that the ethos of 'anything goes' does not necessarily mean that *everything* goes, and that it *is* possible to make judgements between little narratives. Postmodernism entails neither an acceptance nor a rejection of all narratives, but instead an attitude of incredulity, a radical questioning of taken-for-granted beliefs and assumptions, including the assumptions that underpin the entire project of modernist science.

Transposing this argument to the discourse of nursing, I am suggesting that nurses and researchers should adopt an attitude of scepticism towards metanarratives, particularly towards the perceived infallibility of the scientific method. This does not, of course, entail a wholesale rejection of all scientific research findings, but rather a questioning of the rigidly hierarchical relationship between research and practice, what Donald Schön has termed the 'technical rationality' model of professional practice.[4] Statements such as 'the gold standard for evaluating the effectiveness of a [nursing] intervention is the randomized controlled trial',[5] and 'optimal midwifery care can only be achieved through research-based theoretical knowledge and clinical practice'[6] should not be taken at face value; the postmodernist would wish to question the very foundations that underpin such claims. As the original proponents of evidence-based practice themselves acknowledged:

> The proof of the pudding of evidence-based medicine lies in whether patients cared for in this fashion enjoy better health. This proof is no more achievable for the new paradigm [of evidence-based medicine] than it is for the old, for no long-term randomized controlled trials of traditional and evidence-based medical education are likely to be carried out.[7]

Thus, when Phillips condemned new but unfounded (that is, not research-based) ideas in midwifery as 'folklores',[8] she should perhaps have included her own apparently unfounded idea that optimal care can result only from research-based practice. Phillips was plainly not an ironist; she firmly believed that research-based practice is a universal imperative, true for all practitioners at all times. Furthermore, she clearly did not realize the contingency of her position, that research-based practice is but one little narrative with no wider claim to truth than any other little narrative, even by its own standards, since research-based practice is not itself research based.

I raised the possibility at the end of Part I that the rejection of the authority of scientific Method in favour of postmodern ironist methods might be a dangerous move. I hope that I have shown that the danger actually lies in *not* rejecting that authority. To believe that Method always produces the right answers, and to insist that these answers must always be applied to practice, is far more dangerous than the scepticism of the ironist, who accepts the contingency of *all* research findings, regardless of their origins. I also suggested that, by freeing research methods from the tyranny of scientific Method, a far broader range of approaches to data collection (or, as postmodernists would have it, data creation) is possible. The postmodernist, then, does not *reject* the methods of science, but recognizes that they have no automatic claim to truth. More importantly, however, the very act of regarding the metanarrative of Method with scepticism opens the door to a variety of other approaches to research.

Part II of this book offers a number of perspectives on postmodern research, each written by an experienced nurse researcher, and each prefaced with an introduction by myself. The purpose of these introductions is first to place each paper in a slightly wider postmodern context and to clarify some of the words and concepts that are peculiar to postmodernism, and second, to explore and develop some of the author's key ideas in relation to other postmodernist writers. Part II covers a broad spectrum of perspectives, beginning in Chapter Four with Lyotard's original rejection of scientific knowledge in favour of the oral narrative tradition. Chapter Five explores one of the central themes of postmodern research, that of writing, while Chapter Six puts forward the argument for a new postmodern science. The emancipatory feminist perspective is presented in Chapter Seven, and the final chapter in Part II looks at how the postmodern ironist researcher might operate in the real world.

NOTES

1. Blake, W. *Jerusalem*, 1820.
2. Lyotard, J.-F. (1979) *The Postmodern Condition: A Report on Knowledge*, Manchester: Manchester University Press, 1984, p. xxiv.
3. Descartes began his project to 'establish some secure and lasting result in science' (p. 61) by doubting everything. He found, however, that he could not doubt his own existence as a conscious being, since the very act of doubting requires a subject, a 'someone' who doubts. From here, through a series of rather contentious arguments, he concluded that 'from the mere fact that I exist, and have in me some idea of a most perfect being, that is, God, it is clearly demonstrated that God also exists' (p. 90): Descartes, R. (1642) Meditations on first philosophy. In E. Anscombe and P.T. Geach (eds) *Descartes: Philosophical Writings*, London: Open University Press, 1970.
4. Schön, D.A. *The Reflective Practitioner: How Professionals Think in Action*, New York: Basic Books, 1983.
5. French, B. Developing the skills required for evidence-based practice, *Nurse Education Today*, 1998, **18**, 46–51, p. 47.
6. Phillips, R. The need for research-based midwifery practice, *British Journal of Midwifery*, 1994, **2**, 7, 335–8, p. 338.
7. Evidence-Based Medicine Working Group. Evidence-based medicine: a new approach to teaching the practice of medicine, *Journal of the American Medical Association*, 1992, **268**, 17, p. 2424.
8. Phillips, *op. cit.*, p. 336.

CHAPTER FOUR

Postmodern research and the narrative tradition

If it were not for the Poetic or Prophetic Character,
the Philosophic and Experimental would... stand still,
unable to do other than repeat the same dull round over again.[1]

INTRODUCTION

In his seminal work on postmodernism, Lyotard noted that scientific knowledge is a relatively new conception, and contrasted it with 'the preeminence of the narrative form in the formulation of traditional knowledge',[2] in which the usual means of transmission is the story, and more specifically, the oral tradition of storytelling. For Lyotard, then, narrative knowledge, deriving as it does from individual 'little narratives', is a legitimate form of (postmodern) knowledge, and the oral storytelling tradition, as a means of generating and transmitting narrative knowledge, is a legitimate alternative to scientific research. The narrative form is of particular relevance to nursing, which is one of the most recent disciplines to embrace scientific research. Indeed, it is only in the past twenty years or so that scientific knowledge has started to replace narrative knowledge as the academic foundation of nursing theory and practice.

In his early work, Lyotard identified a number of advantages of narrative knowledge over scientific knowledge. First, stories (in the form of myths, legends and apocryphal tales) bestow legitimacy on social institutions or represent positive or negative models. We can see this in nursing, for example in the 'myth' of 'the lady with the lamp', which provides nurses with a blueprint to guide their practice much as the (apocryphal) tales of the life of Jesus provide Christians with a blueprint for moral conduct. In Lyotard's words, such myths allow the discipline 'on the one hand, to define its criteria of competence, and on the other, to evaluate according to those criteria what is performed or can be performed within it'.[3]

Second, the narrative form, unlike the scientific form, lends itself to a great variety of language games. Whereas scientific knowledge favours one particular language game, that of denotation,[4] narrative knowledge can be expressed in a wide variety of forms, including performance and prescription.[5] Scientific knowledge, then, is concerned almost entirely with making statements about what, according to its own criteria, is and is not true. Even Lyotard acknowledged that it is very successful in this enterprise, but it is, nevertheless, a restrictive enterprise that produces a narrow perspective on what counts as knowledge. Narrative, on the other hand, can accommodate a much broader epistemology, and can facilitate the transmission of the 'know-how' necessary for good practice from one generation of nurses to the next, an essential function in disciplines that are predominantly practice centred.

Third, narrative knowledge is inclusive, whereas scientific knowledge is exclusive. The discourse of science simply transmits facts from one who knows to one who does not know, thereby establishing an exclusive club with researchers and academics as knowledge generators on the inside, and practitioners as knowledge users on the outside. It makes no attempt to include the latter in the scientific enterprise; indeed, it actively discourages them from taking part in the process of knowledge generation.[6] In contrast, the narration of a story usually involves a complex network of social rules about who may tell it, who may listen, and who or what qualifies as a legitimate subject of the story. Thus:

> The knowledge transmitted by these narrations is in no way limited to the functions of enunciation; it determines in a single stroke what one must say in order to be heard, what one must listen to in order to speak, and what role one must play... to be the object of a narrative.[7]

Narrative knowledge therefore involves more than simply the transmission of 'the facts' from one who knows to one who does not; a narrative also carries an implicit message about the culture in which it is being told, and 'what is being transmitted through these narratives is a set of pragmatic rules that constitutes the social bond'.[8] A narration without listeners is a pointless exercise (unlike a scientific publication without readers, since it is the act of publication, rather than of being read, that bestows status on the writer), so the listener is just as important in the social act of narration as is the teller.

Finally, whereas the authority of scientific knowledge lies with the sender of the message ('it is true' because I am a scientist, and I will vouch for the authenticity of what I am saying), the authority of narrative knowledge lies in the message itself. As Lyotard pointed out, narratives 'are legitimated by the simple fact that they do what they do'.[9] This position has two important implications. It is, first of all, impossible to judge the validity of either form of knowledge from the basis of the other, since the relevant criteria are different: 'all we can do is gaze in wonderment at the diversity of discursive species, just as we do at the diversity of plant or animal species'.[10] Since narrative knowledge is not concerned with its own legitimation, 'its incomprehension of the problems of scientific discourse is accompanied by a certain tolerance: it approaches such discourse primarily as a variant in the family of narrative cultures'.[11] However, the opposite is not true, since, for the scientific researcher, narrative statements are invalid because they do not conform to the strict criteria of scientific Method. Instead:

> [the researcher] classifies them as belonging to a different mentality: savage, primitive, underdeveloped, backward, alienated, composed of opinions, customs, authority, prejudice, ignorance, ideology. Narratives are fables, myths, legends, fit only for women and children.[12]

Lyotard continued: 'This unequal relationship is an intrinsic effect of the rules specific to each game. We all know its symptoms. *It is the entire history of cultural imperialism from the dawn of Western civilization*'.[13] We can see this effect at work on the discourse of nursing, which has, until recently, been viewed by the scientific community as (to borrow Lyotard's words) 'primitive, underdeveloped, backward... composed of opinions, customs, authority, prejudice, ignorance, ideology... fit only for women...', in other words, as a prime candidate for scientific cultural imperialism. Consequently, science has presented itself as a 'civilizing influence' in suppressing the oral tradition of nursing in favour of a research-based approach that 'de-emphasizes intuition, unsystematic clinical experience and pathophysiologic rationale as sufficient grounds for clinical decision making and stresses the examination of evidence from clinical research'.[14] From this perspective, then, the oral narrative does not even qualify as research, and is relegated to the lowest position in the hierarchy of nursing knowledge. The danger is, however, that the suppression of the narrative form is accompanied by the suppression of nursing 'know-how' and tacit knowledge, what Benner[15] has referred to as intuitive expertise.

KIM WALKER ON THE 'POETICS AND POLITICS OF ORALITY'

The following discussion by Walker is an attempt to redress the balance by arguing that nursing *must* retain and develop its oral culture, that 'practice is given voice in the narrative fragments of daily conversation'.[16] But he goes further: nursing does not merely *have* an oral culture, nursing *is* an oral culture. However, this culture clashes with the scientific culture that has recently been imposed from outside. Thus, as Walker points out, it is a culture 'in which nurses currently struggle with some fundamental contradictions in the ways we attempt to organize and make sense of our lives as clinicians'. The contradictions, of course, arise from what amounts to a culture clash between the oral tradition of nursing practice and the imposed culture of science and the scientific method.

Walker is very alert to Lyotard's ideas about science as a form of cultural imperialism, and argues that in order to fight it off, nursing must mobilize all of its forces. It is not enough merely for practitioners to continue to uphold the oral tradition in the face of ever more pressure for written documentation, as in Walker's example of the oral versus the written handover. Instead, he wishes to see the entire profession throw its academic and political weight behind narrativity, which, he argues, 'can constitute a mode of research' in its own right. Narrativity is, however, more than just another research method: it is 'a methodological imperative'[17] that enables us 'to ask critical questions of the significant and (seemingly) inconsequential moments of our histories and of the ways those histories inform and inflect our individual and collective understandings as nurses'.

For Walker, there are a number of reasons why the oral tradition should be associated with the postmodern turn. First, there is the timely breakdown of the scientific discourse, what he terms (borrowing from Lather) the 'twilight of modernity'. Thus, 'in a strategic reappropriation of such a moment', we must 'be mobilized and radicalized by the new order of things in which certainty collides with ambiguity and totalities splinter into fragments'. This, of course, involves a scepticism towards the metanarrative of Method in favour of 'the archives of a culture', in which individual little narratives 'slowly accrue to become a culture's common sense and folklore, its theories and knowledge'.[18]

Second, Walker concurs with Lyotard about the pre-eminence of language and language games in the narrative turn. Thus, whereas, for Walker, the aim of science is to *describe* an existing reality, 'our lives and experiences are not merely reflected in stories; they are instead, actually *created* by and through them' (emphasis added); and more explicitly, 'I think of language as rather more generative of what we loosely call "reality" than as merely descriptive of such a possible thing.' He then goes on to describe in some detail the 'codes and forms' that the language game of narrative draws upon in order to convey its messages, and, following the work of Hillis Miller, identifies:

- that narratives need to be situated with/in language
- that they require a 'cast' of people/actors
- that they rely on a patterning or repetition of key elements (for example, metaphors) in a 'narrative rhythm'
- that, most importantly, they require a plot for order and orientation.

It could be argued that Walker has perhaps not gone far enough here, that what he is advocating is a structuralist interpretation rather than a post-structuralist or postmodernist one. Thus, he is concerned to explain how the listener is able to share and understand the codes and forms of the narrator, with how the meaning given to a story by the teller is able to be accurately transmitted, rather than with Barthes' suggestion that there is no single meaning, and that 'the birth of the reader must be at the cost of the death of the Author'.[19] However, Walker should perhaps be commended for not expecting nursing to run before it can walk. Perhaps we need to come to terms with the notion of the narrative as a legitimate form of research and transmitter of knowledge before we take the argument to its (for some) logical conclusion; we must first construct the discourse of narrative knowledge before we attempt to deconstruct it.

Having established a case for narrativity, Walker then turns his attention to the dual focus of his title: the poetics and politics of the oral tradition. He argues that nursing is a culture in Giroux's sense of the term as a site of struggle over 'the representation of lived experiences, material artifacts and practices forged in the unequal dialectic relations that given groups establish within a given society at a particular point in time'.[20] In the case of nursing, Walker interprets this as the struggle between the oral tradition of practitioners and the written tradition of nurse leaders and academics, a struggle in which the oral is at a clear disadvantage with respect to the written.[21] The difficulty in attempting to assert the oral tradition of narrativity is that the (scientific) language game of nursing largely precludes discussions of this kind; narrative knowledge simply does not count.[22] Thus, while 'such contradictions continue to shape nursing culture', these contradictions remain largely untheorized. The narrative tradition is therefore faced with a dual problem: not only has the oral tradition been suppressed, but also it has been so 'written out' of the discourse of nursing that we can now only discuss it meaningfully from within the language game of science.

Walker's solution to this dilemma is not to attempt the difficult (if not impossible) task of 'talking up' narrativity as a form of scientific discourse, but instead to challenge the scientific hegemony[23] head on. Following Gramsci, then, Walker argues for a 'counter-hegemony', specifically for 'the poetic moment as a counter-hegemonic technique of sensibility', a strategy to oppose the hegemony of empirical research and the written word. There is no point in attempting to argue for the 'poetic moment' in the language (game) of science. Instead, like Rorty, we must simply describe the world from the perspective of our own language game and in our own language, and hope that it will prove tempting to others. Thus, Walker offers a poem as a means of articulating the 'trivial, ordinary and routine' of everyday practice, indeed as a structure through which we can accumulate and express our cultural knowledge and critical procedures. Storytelling becomes a research method that can 'valorize the spoken and heard over the seen and observed'; indeed, it is *the* research method, since all empirical observation must be transformed and translated into language during the process of data collection. Thus, 'what we can learn about ourselves and our world is so much more reliant on how we hear and listen to ourselves... than what we might deduce otherwise, from our observations'.

Having explicated the epistemological side of his project as a 'poetics of experience', Walker now turns his attention to the political side, and more precisely, to a 'politics of desire', a term borrowed from the postmodernist philosophers Deleuze and Guattari. For Walker, the politics of desire has influenced the nursing profession in a negative way, as 'a form of restraint rather than release'. In its negative form, desire stems from a lack of what others have and a yearning to be like others;[24] in the case of nurses, to be like the 'great scientists and medical/administrative leaders of health care... to the point that their own needs and demands as women and as health care workers have been subjugated and subjected to the will of those dominant "others"'. From this perspective, the replacement of the traditional epistemology of narrativity with the epistemology of science and the scientific method can be seen as an attempt to fill the 'hole' of desire.

However, Walker urges us to subscribe not to this version of desire as a lack, but to a positive version of desire as 'a form of dreaming, of searching for something beyond ourselves', which 'imagines another order of things altogether'. This other order of things is located in 'the socially constructed "reality" that the culture of nursing is in a state of vertiginous flux... precarious and unstable despite "others" attempts to create an illusion of fixity and security'. Thus, the politics of desire (in its positive sense) opposes those 'others' (mainly American nurse theorists) who attempt to foster the illusion of nursing as a 'monolithic and stable structure', and who are motivated by the lack (the negative meaning of the term desire) of a hard scientific basis for nursing. We thus cannot separate the poetics and the politics of nursing; the politics of desire deconstructs the metanarrative built by the 'great' nursing theorists, and the poetics of experience offers a framework of narrative knowledge with which to replace it. For Walker, then, 'to do research and bravely take the postmodern turn, [and here he quotes Spanos] "is to move into the space of deconstructing/deconstructive inquiry, to tell stories that end in neither comprehended knowledge nor incapacitating textual undecidibility"'.

Nursing, narrativity and research: towards a poetics and politics of orality[25]

Kim Walker

ENTERING THE 'FIELD'

When was the last time you recollected a riotously funny mishap in which you were implicated, or told of a genuinely moving experience in your life as a nurse? How often have you found yourself telling a story of a particularly difficult day at work, or perhaps of some especially tragic moment in a patient's life, only to find yourself wondering if your audience knows just exactly what it is that you're talking about?

As nurses, we compile in a life of practice, an incredible chronicle of experience that comes to expression in the everyday stories we share over the dinner table, in the wee small hours of night duty and over numerous cups of coffee at our friends' houses. Have you ever mused over what it might be like to somehow capture something of that vast and messy thing called 'practice' so that a permanent record could be accumulated for reflection, analysis, theorizing – a sort of record of the present as history?

What I hope to do here is create a space in which nurses might like to (re)think their relation to their practice, particularly as that practice is given voice in the narrative fragments of daily conversation. What I want to suggest is that such 'narrative rememberings'[26] can constitute a mode of research of and for our culture, because it seems to me that we know very little of what it is that we do, let alone how and why we might do what we do in the ways that we do.

Indulging in some theoretical reflections on the relationship between narrative structures, language, and the ways we are able to make sense of the world, I lay bare the 'ground' of my argument. I suggest that narrative can be regarded as both a research method as well as a methodological imperative for better understanding of the practices and languages which shape us as nurses, as we in turn shape those practices and languages.

To do this work, nursing must be theorized as a culture. Indeed it must be thought of primarily as an 'oral' culture; one in which nurses currently struggle with some fundamental contradictions in the ways we attempt to organize and make sense of our lives as clinicians. Thinking of nursing as a culture allows us to ask critical questions of the significant and (seemingly) inconsequential moments of our histories and of the ways those histories inform and inflect our individual and collective understandings as nurses.

It seems to me then, that the 'politics of desire' which has informed nurses' individual and collective understandings of what constitutes 'good' research must be rethought. I engage in an extremely partial and provisional critique of the ways we have thought of research in nursing through a specific 'frame of constructed visibility'[27] called the 'modern'. I argue how, in the 'twilight of modernity',[28] we might make research spaces for ourselves which contest those 'received' understandings of what constitutes good research, and set up research processes in and through which we can begin to 'tell nursing like it is' by appropriating narratives of everyday life in clinical practice.

In bringing together nursing and its narratives of practice as a technology of research, we can anticipate a poetics and politics of orality, ever mindful that in a culture composed and ceaselessly recomposed with every utterance, in each fragment of a narrative is contained something which both belongs yet is borrowed, coheres yet conflicts with our own and someone else's reality. A narrative history, at once seemingly singular and monolithic, becomes plural and fragile. Nurses talk. They tell their lives and speak their bodies – words create meanings from desire and as they dredge sedimented knowledges in the 'will to understand' their lives, nurses' narrative rememberings become the archives of a culture. Words construct identities in their passing. Nurses share stories among themselves and, in the late-night-early-morning-all-day conversations, are spun the myths and fables, those fantasies and fictions which slowly accrue to become a culture's common sense and folklore, its theories and knowledge.

The stories we share daily harbour the dramatic and mundane, the obvious and the arcane, the general and the specific of our culture. The narrative structures which inhere in those fragile chains of spoken words we come to know as 'dialogue', in all that comes to language, are perhaps the most central structures in the sense making activities through which we mediate and negotiate the pressing contingencies and necessities of everyday life as a nurse. Our lives and experiences are not merely reflected in stories; they are instead, actually created by and through them.

ORALITY, NARRATIVE, DIALOGUE – THE SEEMINGLY REMOTE STRUCTURES OF EVERYDAY LIFE

Just what might these narrative structures to which I refer be, and why might they be so important? How might they work to help us bring to life research methodologies forged in relations of collaboration, dialogue and storytelling? In the philosophical position which currently informs my thinking, I think of language as rather more generative of what we loosely call 'reality' than as merely descriptive of such a possible thing. And if this is the case, then it must follow that *the ways in which we use language are utterly pivotal*, if we think of one of life's most significant tasks – making sense of a life – in terms of the meanings we can derive from our experiences in the world as nurses. As J. Hillis Miller, a prominent literary theorist, puts it:

> We give experience a form and a meaning, a linear order with a shapely beginning, middle, end, and a central theme. The human capacity to tell stories is one way men and women collectively build a significant and orderly world around themselves. With fictions we investigate, perhaps invent, the meaning of human life.[29]

Narratives and their function have preoccupied the work of scholars working in the 'human sciences' for the last seventy years or so. Coming at the centrality of narrative in human existence a little from behind, consider the process of reading. Robert Scholes tells us:

> We can only understand a story if we have read enough other stories to understand the elements of narrative coding. Our first stories are told or read to us by our parents, or other parental figures, who explain the codes as they go. The ideal reader shares the author's codes and is able to process the text without confusion or delay. Such a reader constructs a whole world for us from a few indications, fills in gaps, makes temporal correlations... all without hesitation or difficulty.[30]

How might this be possible, for surely it is a remarkable thing to be able to do? It is so remarkable, in fact, that such a complex and sophisticated act of simultaneously reading, interpreting, deconstructing, reconstructing and telling, has assumed a sort of 'naturalness' by the time we are not very old at all. Indeed if 'narrating is a unique language-game' and a language-game 'is a part of an activity or form of life',[31] then to what rules does such a game conform? What codes and forms must a narrative draw upon in order that it work in the ways to which I have been attesting?

It seems that the narrative structures most fundamental to the ways in which we are able to ascribe meaningful (which is to say, sufficiently coherent, accessible and believable) interpretations to our experiences, are relatively few. 'There must be, first of all, an initial situation, a sequence leading to a change or reversal of that situation, and a revelation made possible by the [change or] reversal of that situation'.[32] When we consider the context specificity of all nursing practice, its profoundly situated, yet uncertain and ever changing nature, then it is not difficult to imagine that these formative agents of the narrative activities in which we daily engage, abound. Indeed, as human agents we always find ourselves in a situation.[33] Our world only has meaning because we live in the world, 'always already' with and in language, as we are 'speaking subjects'[34] for whom the meaning of our experiences is only ever constituted in the languages we have at our disposal. Language, as Martin Heidegger puts it so elegantly, is 'the house of being'.[35] That 'house' is always situated in a larger terrain, the geography of the social and cultural world we inhabit with every moment of our conscious existence.

But if narratives need a situation which can be reversed or changed and some new insight be generated through the process of such a change or reversal, then they also need a character, or 'some personification whereby [a] character is created out of signs',[36] as for example, in the descriptions of various actors on the page of a novel, or in the 'modulated sounds in the air in an oral narrative'.[37] For our world only matters to us because we live in the world with others.[38] The 'other' is the necessity without which we cannot meaningfully exist. All our stories of and in the world are peopled stories. They would barely be worth telling if they weren't. And consider that even when we tell a story about a 'thing', there is always an actor, even if that actor is ourselves or the listener! Indeed, it is not possible to tell a story without, in some way, presupposing an 'other' because the act of telling a story is itself thoroughly dialogical. It is a narrating, a telling *to* or *for* or *about* or *of* ourselves, each other and the world of which we are not merely a part, but a world without which we would not be at all.

The third structure inherent in the narrative moment insists that storytelling relies on some 'patterning or repetition of key elements',[39] for example, certain figures of speech or particular metaphors or specific complex words (such as words with more than one obvious meaning). Or to put it another way, there must be a sort of narrative rhythm which modulates (which is to say, regulates or adapts to the circumstances) that figure of speech, metaphor or complex word. Such things abound in our stories, but rarely do they appear to our conscious awareness. Metaphor, for example, is so ubiquitous as to assume a transparency alarming in its audacity, beguiling in its unassuming complexity. Metaphors, as Schrag[40] comments so accurately, do not simply adorn our understandings, they actually carry them.

Consider the 'journey' metaphor I have invoked in the construction of my argument, or the 'hands on' metaphor of our culture[41] which calls up such potent meanings for us. These metaphors so thoroughly imbue our vernacular that we cease even to think of them as metaphors. They impart a narrative rhythm to our storytelling events by returning the listener to the impulse each metaphor or figure of speech employs to sustain its particular figurative 'effect'. In the instance of the 'journey' metaphor for example, we are, as narrator/listeners, caught simultaneously in the imagery of travel as we are carried by the 'travel' of the story itself. Such a metaphor becomes an orienting device and at the same time it propels the narrator/listener forward in the narrative encounter through its anticipation and repetition (in much the same way the regular beat and melody of music does).

But the most important structure on which narrative turns is, of course, that of plot. This is not just to imagine a beginning, middle and an end to a story. For as Paul Ricoeur tells us, 'there is no story unless our attention is held in suspense by a thousand contingencies'.[42] Stories, as I intimated above, are always a shared activity, and it is in the dialogical act of sharing a story that the narrative structures of situation, character and rhythm come to life through that most central element of plot. Plot draws together other rudiments of narrative such as place, space and time. It is through the orienting and dynamic interaction of each of these elements that plot is woven and, in Michel de Certeau's words, 'stories [are able to] traverse and organize places; they select and link places together making sentences and itineraries out of them'.[43] This concatenation of narrative structures weaves for the human agent a world in which:

> it is language itself, narratives, the stories we tell each other, that tends towards becoming what Derrida terms the factor of truth... a sense of reality which is not something that can be reduced to... reason, history, [or] progress... but is rather something that becomes, that emerges through difference, through specificity, through dialogue, through our languages and histories; that is, in the insistent intercourse of the world.[44]

Narratives forge their significance for us as nurses in the articulation of everyday practices, 'where to name and describe is both an act of appropriation and an expression of dexterity, the exercise of know-how or common sense knowledge'.[45] Each of these narrative structures underscores how 'the story plays a decisive role [in human existence]'. It 'describes', but 'every description is more than a fixation', it is 'a culturally creative act'.[46]

NURSING AS 'ORAL' CULTURE: A CULTURE OF CONTRADICTIONS

It seems to me that if we recognize the 'narrativity' of everyday life, then we also need to think of nursing as a culture – in the sense that it constitutes a site of struggle over the 'representation of lived experiences, material artifacts and practices forged in the unequal dialectical relations that different groups establish within a given society at a particular point in time'.[47]

In Giroux's terms then, thinking of nursing as a culture requires us to understand simultaneously, for example, the lived experiences of clinical nurses, the material artifacts produced and consumed by nurse scholars, and the practices of nurse administrators as 'representing' themselves and struggling to coexist in a set of inherently unequal relations. They are 'representations' moreover, that are always maintained by nurses in a sort of tension between which of them more accurately reflects (or more properly, constructs) the culture of nursing at any specific moment in history.

Building on Giroux's notion of a culture as a 'form of production' and a site of struggle, I also follow Annette Street, who has argued persuasively that clinical nursing is constituted primarily as an oral culture. 'The culture of clinical nursing [she tells us] is an uncharted map of nursing care in which the values of clinical nurses are taken for granted and therefore, are not always evident in the values espoused by nursing leaders'.[48] The saliency of Street's work for us can, in the context of my discussion here, be theorized in:

> the ways in which the oral basis of nursing culture causes nurses to continue to be oppressed because they are unable to move from individualism to collaboration, they are unable to document their clinical knowledge and practice for reflection and critique, and they are unable to challenge the power base of the medical and administrative cultures articulated and perpetuated through means of written communication.[49]

Street's idea that an oral culture somehow contributes to the ways in which we both enact and perpetually re-enact the conditions of our domination is a significant one. If, as I have been working to argue, with every story, with every 'culturally creative act', as de Certeau would say, something is made and simultaneously lost, then in a culture which relies heavily on the oral transmission of knowledge and understandings, what can be said, to whom and about what, becomes an issue of centrality for research. I have alluded to how contradictions constitute our worlds in particular ways. Let me amplify this suggestion.

Consider the way nurse administrators 'expend a great deal of energy directed at the development of the recording skills and practices of clinical nurses'.[50] Documentation, in the late 1980s, became the buzz word for clinical nurses. Obsessive attention was paid to what we wrote, and more particularly, to how we wrote. Nursing care plans were seen as the exemplar of good practice and clinicians were exhorted not only to write them up within twenty-four hours of a patient's admission, but then to keep them scrupulously up to date. But such a project, I argue, was doomed to failure because the administrators failed to recognize that while they implored clinical nurses to document and keep records of what, when and how they did their work, 'at the same time they supported and maintained the oral culture of nursing through structural practices such as the oral handover and the double shift time'. Clinical nurses rightly asked themselves: 'why bother to write it all down when I'm going to "tell" all my nursing care in much more detail during the handover?' The tension engendered by administrators and clinicians, the latter who value *speaking* the world and the former whose rhetoric values *writing* that very same world, arises from a profound conflict of interests. Bureaucratic discourses privilege the rational, the ordered and the stable. Clinical discourses on the other hand, are produced from the institutional and power/knowledge relations of the contingent world of practice, which valorize the relative immediacy, incoherence and instability of that practice world.

Such contradictions continue to shape nursing culture because these potent forces, these 'discourses' which shape how we think into how we actually act as nurses, have remained largely untheorized until recently. It is the project of uncovering such forces that urges nursing scholars to seek ever more persuasive and adequate explanations for *why we do what we do the way we do*. 'Telling' the culture of nursing 'like it is' can be one such way of better locating the structures and relations which not only maintain the cultural practices we engage daily, but more pertinently, of thinking around how we might engage some of them differently.

THE POETIC MOMENT AS A COUNTER-HEGEMONIC TECHNIQUE OF SENSIBILITY

In order to amplify my claims about the primacy of the oral in nursing, I will deflect my line of thought in a slightly different direction now. In a poetics of embodiment (a languaged form that speaks our bodies and identities at one and the same moment) a schooldays friend captured an infinitesimal moment in her experience as nurse; one of those precarious realities which pass us stealthily, silently slipping into the storehouse of memories seldom recalled and little valued:

> i remember
> on afternoonshift
> how i stroked
> my own passion
> into some old lady's
> unsunned
> flabby back
> concentrating
> in the afterdinner
> hotwash
> on stupefying
> the sick old body
> into fragile
> comfort
> with these gentle
> insistent
> attentions[51]

Janet, my school-friend, 'speaks' and 'narrates' herself as 'nurse', as a young woman who found herself inserted in a culture not of her making, a culture beguiling in its intricacy and diversity, alarming in its violence and perversity. After her training, Janet never really worked as a registered nurse. It is thus ever more remarkable that she 'remembers', and thus retraces a tiny, but clearly significant detail from her life as a student of nursing through these poetic fragments, these narrative rememberings of a life once lived, now brought to eloquent expression. For undoubtedly, the three years spent learning to be a nurse etched something of their materiality on and into her identity as a woman. And in these words is caught a moment we all know and have shared. Such an elegantly simple chain of signifiers vivifies and incarnates the work we do, which is often dismissed and demeaned as trivial, ordinary and routine. But it is work only some care to do; few others could or would care to do. This poem's occult sensuality and disarming honesty evokes the sad banality and poignant insignificance of much of our work. Yet Janet's ephemeral lyric of a culture spoken creates a space into which each of us who are nurses, can temporarily insert ourselves; it is exactly that space 'where to name and describe is both an act of appropriation and an expression of dexterity, the exercise of know-how or commonsense knowledge'[52] which I mentioned earlier. It is in such an 'articulation of everyday activities'[53] through which narratives as 'descriptions' become 'more than a fixation... [they become, as Michel de Certeau told us] a culturally creative act'.[54]

But the 'world', as I hinted earlier, which is created through narration is 'not a secure world, it only lasts as long as the story is remembered and every time it is retold the world is created anew'.[55] Janet's 'creative act' recreates a world in its telling and our world can become

> a certain world because it is based on the narrative processes by which we describe the world to ourselves in our own terms to our own satisfaction, enabling us to manipulate that world and to move around in it.[56]

Thus, a poetics of experience brings to language through the process of writing, something on which we can graft 'an open, ever-changing theoretical structure by which to order both our cultural knowledge and our critical procedures'.

All of which is not to suggest that nurses take up writing poetry (although perhaps it would be not such a bad thing that they did). Rather, I am coming at the value, utility and significance of story-telling as a research method that is inscribed within methodological frameworks such as ethnography and action research. They are research frameworks which, despite their claims to do otherwise, actually valorize the spoken and heard over the seen and observed. The research imperative in both of these methodological 'frames of constructed visibility',[57] while ostensibly skewed toward the seen and observed, invariably *transforms* and *translates* 'empirical' data into language to be read and heard. My contention here is that 'seeing is always mediated by saying'.[58] What we can learn about ourselves and our world is so much more reliant on how we hear and listen to ourselves and our world than what we might deduce otherwise, from our observations (which will ultimately be made sense of through the linguistic processes we have available to us).

THE POLITICS OF DESIRE: MOVING BEYOND THE TYRANNY OF CONVENTIONAL RESEARCH DESIGN

The project of 'telling it like it is' is forged in a politics of desire; a politics in which a position of radical critique is assumed by she who chooses to tell and write her story(s). A politics of desire both preempts and exceeds the demands of the self, its social construction and its specific temporal location. I believe that a particular form of the politics of desire, in which a culture's history(s) becomes a form of restraint rather than release, has operated since the birth of the modern nurse in the mid 19th century. The modes of desire which nursing has submitted itself to for the last 150 years have been modes formed in our individual and collective unconscious needs to be like the 'other', to have what it is the 'other' has and which makes him legitimate and successful. Nurses' sense of themselves has been locked into 'modes of desire'[59] in which the 'other' is always white, male and endowed with certain knowledges; knowledges which inscribe authority, influence and privilege on the bodies of those who claim to possess them. These men have been the great scientists and medical/administrative leaders of health care, they have been omnipotent 'others' whose 'will to power' has placed them beyond reproach, almost beyond desire itself. Nurses have made a fetish of this seductive 'other' to the point that their own needs and demands as women and as health care workers have been subjugated and subjected to the will of those dominant 'others'. In the process, nurses' needs and demands have been stifled and suppressed.

But desire is something altogether different from need and demand. Desire lies on the other side of need; it 'emerges when satisfaction of need is not enough, where there is a doubt or a gap which cannot be closed'.[60] That 'gap which cannot be closed' can be found in the cultural space produced through the irreconcilable differences we embody as members of a social group whose identities will always be ascribed less worth than those dominant 'others' I mentioned above. It is a 'gap' formed in the margins, an 'in between' space of the not-quite-here, not-quite-there. The 'demand' that nurses be recognized as equals to those dominant 'others' will never be satisfied and this will push nurses to other demands such as those for better pay and better material conditions in which to do their work. bell hooks describes this process as a sort of 'yearning', a deeply felt longing to be 'like' the other.[61]

Rather than subscribe to this version of desire as 'lack' (which is rather more constraining than enlivening for us), we can (re)think desire as it is a 'form of dreaming, of searching for something beyond ourselves'[62] (but *not* in the sense of searching for something which someone else has, that we too must have). This is a form of desire that imagines another order of things altogether. And it is in such a 'form of dreaming' that a new politics of desire must be situated and from which its field of force must emanate. The primary technology through which a new politics of desire must be mobilized can be located in the socially constructed 'reality' that the culture of nursing is in a state of vertiginous flux. It is precarious and unstable despite 'others' attempts to create an illusion of fixity and security.

The 'others' to whom I refer here are, of course, the eminent nurse theorists whose writings now form an enormous repository of scholarship on the 'nature' of nursing and its work. These women have worked tirelessly over the last several decades to produce a body of evidence that testifies to nursing's worth in the hierarchy of (scientific) knowledge. Only recently have nurses in spaces 'other' to those colonized by the North American icons of nursing's intellectual work begun to critique the production of such knowledge. In my own[63] and others' work,[64] can be heard the rumblings of a critique that dares to suggest that perhaps we have been misguided and deluded in our search for an 'Archimedean point',[65] a place on which to anchor our sense of ourselves and our work that will not move; a place that will speak its name with the same clarity and resolution that we have heard in those who call themselves 'scientist' or 'philosopher'. As I hope is becoming apparent, the culture of nursing and the knowledges and practices which both form and are formed with/in its ever permeable boundaries can no longer be seen as if they constituted a monolithic and stable structure.

'Telling' the culture of nursing 'like it is' can be thought of then, as a political topology, a deconstructive strategy, and a process of critique in which:

> critique is not a matter of saying that things are not right as they are. It is a matter of pointing out on what kinds of assumptions, what kinds of familiar, unchallenged, uncontested modes of thought the practices that we accept rest.[66]

If a postmodern politics of desire in and from which we might care to imagine a new place to 'speak' ourselves as nurses must always be 'lived out in historically and culturally specific forms,[67] then the crumbling of the twentieth century marks a historically specific juncture for nursing from which we must now confront the 'effects' in our culture of those dominant 'regimes of truth'[68] which have held us captive for so long.

A SPACE TO (RE)CREATE OUR HISTORIES: TAKING THE
POSTMODERN TURN

As I move this text toward its inevitable point of closure, I want, in a
deliberately destabilizing strategy, to make explicit the space from
which my thoughts and words have issued. The primacy of language
as 'constructing' of reality, of narrative as a culturally creative act, and
the inherently dialogical nature of our experiences which I have
spoken about in detail here, owe the possibility of their expression as
central organizing principles in making sense of a life, to the postmodern turn.

Indeed, it is the view of an increasing number in the academy of the
late twentieth century that we are confronted with:

> a most uncomfortable form of intellectual vertigo to which appropriate
> responses are not clear. It is increasingly difficult even to begin to know
> how to comprehend what we are thinking and experiencing.[69]

Flax speaks, of course, of that contentious yet undeniable cultural
shift in the academy which is informed by poststructural theories of,
among other things, knowledge, identity, language, gender and
power. Through the twilight of modernity some of us glimpse the
dawning of postmodernity. If we are not to be paralysed by the effects
of such a disquieting moment we must instead, I believe, in a strategic
re-appropriation of such a moment, be mobilized and radicalized by
the new order of things in which certainty collides with ambiguity
and totalities splinter into fragments; where truth is no longer
singular but plural and nonoppositional forms of difference are not
merely celebrated, but are actually grafted onto a politics of identity
and location in which, as nurses, we come to 'make a definite distinction between that marginality which is imposed by oppressive structures and that marginality one chooses as a site of resistance – as [a]
location of radical openness and possibility'.[70]

This would be an order of things suspicious of 'grand narratives'[71]
such as science, phenomenology, Marxism or capitalism; stories that
attempt to tell us how to live our lives. It would be a 'space of radical
openness and possibility' in which identities are spoken from within a
politics of difference and experience ever attentive to the ways in which
gender, age, race, class and sexual preference (among others) position
each of us precariously on sites of struggle over how best to interpret
our lives.

Taking up a postmodern 'sensibility' as I am suggesting, urges us, as
researchers, to effect a politics of difference in and through which we

can begin to 'textualize identities at their most vulnerable moments, to speak about and for individuals by juxtaposing their words with [our] own, [and thus]... dramatize the ordinary days that make time seem like no time at all'.[72] Indeed, to do research and bravely take the postmodern turn, 'is to move into the space of deconstructing/deconstructive inquiry, to tell stories that end in neither comprehended knowledge nor incapacitating textual undecidibility'.[73] It is, furthermore, to acknowledge that:

> it is the potential for social action in language interactions, the sheer desire to critique and change an unsatisfying social reality, that brings people to speech and writing. It is on this promise that language is or can be liberating... that we produce as well as reproduce culture in speech and writing.

NOTES

1. Blake, W. *There is No Natural Religion*, 1788.
2. Lyotard, J.-F. (1979) *The Postmodern Condition: A Report on Knowledge*, Manchester: Manchester University Press, 1984.
3. *Ibid.*, p. 20.
4. Denotative utterances are essentially utterances of truth and falsehood, for example, 'this is the best way of dressing a wound'.
5. Performative utterances are utterances which produce that which is uttered; for example, the very act of saying 'the exam has now started' actually starts the exam. Prescriptive utterances are utterances which demand something of someone, for example, 'do it like this'.
6. For example, the Department of Health has asserted that 'research, done properly, is a highly professional and specialist activity and not suited to every practitioner': Department of Health *The Nursing and Therapy Professions' Contribution to Health Services Research and Development*. London: DoH, 1995.
7. Lyotard, *op. cit.*, p. 21.
8. *Ibid.*, p. 21.
9. *Ibid.*, p. 23.
10. *Ibid.*, p. 26.
11. *Ibid.*, p. 27.
12. *Ibid.*, p. 27.
13. *Ibid.*, p. 27, emphasis added.
14. Evidence-Based Medicine Working Group. Evidence-based medicine: a new approach to teaching the practice of medicine, *Journal of the American Medical Association*, 1992, **268**, 17, p. 2420.
15. Benner, P. *From Novice to Expert*, Menlo Park, CA: Addison-Wesley, 1984.

16. All unreferenced quotations are from Walker's section in this chapter.

17. In other words, it is urgent or essential.

18. It is, perhaps, worth pointing out that this is *precisely* the mentality which science wishes to be rid of, and which Lyotard characterized (from the perspective of science) as 'savage, primitive, underdeveloped, backward, alienated, composed of opinions, customs, authority, prejudice, ignorance, ideology', and ultimately 'fit only for women and children': Lyotard, *op. cit.*, p. 27.

19. Barthes, R. (1968) The death of the author. In R. Barthes *Image Music Text*, S. Heath (trans.), London: Fontana, 1977, p. 148. See Chapter 2 of this book for a fuller discussion of Barthes and post-structuralism.

20. Giroux, H. Introduction. In P. Freire *The Politics of Education: Culture, Power and Liberation*, D. Macedo (trans.), Basingstoke: Macmillan, 1985, p. xxi.

21. It is interesting to contrast this view with Derrida's opposing notion of 'logocentrism', which is not only 'the exclusion or abasement of writing', but also extends to the spoken word 'the granting of authority to a science which is held to be the model for all the so-called sciences of man' (p. 102). Thus, at least in the human sciences, writing has been relegated to merely the mechanical representation of the spoken word. Later in the same work, Derrida conflates the prejudice of logocentrism (the dominance of the spoken word) with that of phalocentrism (the dominance of male culture) into the single word 'phalogocentrism'. Derrida, J. (1967) *Of Grammatology*, G.C. Spivak (trans.), Baltimore: John Hopkins University Press, 1974.

22. This is a good example of Lyotard's notion of the *differend*, in which claims between competing language games are judged according to the standards of one of them, to the disadvantage of the other. Lyotard, J.-F. *The Differend: Phrases in Dispute*, Minneapolis: University of Minnesota Press, 1988.

23. That is, science as cultural authority (and hence power).

24. Walker is, perhaps, making reference to Lacan's argument that desire is a 'hole' that can only be filled by the desire of another.

25. First published in *Contemporary Nurse*, 1995, **4**, 156–63.

26. De Concini, B. *Narrative Remembering*, Lanham: University of America Press, 1990.

27. Lather, P. 'The Politics and Ethics of Feminist Research: Researching the Lives of Women with AIDS', Draft of an address prepared for the Ethnography and Education Research Forum, Philadelphia, PA, 1993.

28. Lather, P. *Getting Smart... Feminist Research and Pedagogy with/in the Postmodern*, London: Routledge, 1991.

29. Hillis-Miller, J. Narrative. In F. Lentdcchia and T. McLaughlin (eds) *Critical Terms for Literary Study*, Chicago: University of Chicago Press, 1990, p. 69.

30. Scholes, R. *Textual Power: Literary Theory and the Teaching of English*, New Haven: Yale University Press, 1985.

31. Ricouer, P. *Hermeneutics and the Human Sciences*, J.B. Thompson (ed.), Cambridge: Cambridge University Press, 1981, p. 274.

32. Hillis Miller, *op. cit.*, p. 75.

33. Heidegger, M. *Being and Time*, J. Macquarie and E. Robinson (trans.), Oxford: Basil Blackwell, 1962.

34. Kristeva, J. *Desire in Language: A Semiotic Approach to Art and Literature*, L.S. Roudiez (trans.), New York: University of Columbia Press, 1980. Weedon, C. *Feminist Practice and Poststructuralist Theory*, Oxford: Basil Blackwell, 1987.

35. Heidegger, M. *Poetry, Language, Thought*, A. Hofstadter (trans.), New York: Harper & Row, 1971.

36. Hillis Miller, *op. cit.*, p. 75.

37. *Ibid.*, p. 75.

38. Heidegger, 1962, *op. cit.*

39. Hillis Miller, *op. cit.*, p. 75.

40. Schrag, C.O. *Communicative Praxis and the Space of Subjectivity*, Bloomington: Indiana University Press, 1986.

41. Walker, K. On What it Might Mean To Be a Nurse: A Discursive Ethnography, Unpublished doctoral dissertation, Melbourne: La Trobe University, 1993.

42. Ricouer, *op. cit.*, p. 277.

43. Revill, G. Reading Rosehill Community, identity and inner-city Derby. In G. Revill, *Place and the Politics of Identity*, London: Routledge, 1993, p. 130.

44. Chambers, I. *Border Dialogues: Journeys in Postmodernity*, London: Routledge, 1990, pp. 4–5.

45. Revill, *op. cit.*, p. 130.

46. de Certeau, M. *The Practice of Everyday Life*, Berkeley: University of California Press, 1984, p. 123.

47. Giroux, H. Introduction. In P. Freire *The Politics of Education: Culture, Power and Liberation*, D. Macedo (trans.), Basingstoke: Macmillan, 1985, p. xxi.

48. Street, A. *Inside Nursing: A Critical Ethnography of Nursing*, New York: State University of New York Press, 1992, p. 267.

49. *Ibid.*, p. 267.

50. *Ibid.*, p. 268.

51. Charman, J. *2 Deaths In 1 Night*, Auckland: New Women's Press, 1987.

52. Revill, *op. cit.*, p. 130.

53. *Ibid.*, p. 130.

54. de Certeau, cited in Revill, *ibid.*, p. 130.

55. *Ibid.*, p. 130.

56. *Ibid.*, p. 130.

57. Lather, *op. cit.*, 1993.

58. Tyler, S. *The Unspeakable: Discourse, Dialogue and Rhetoric in the Postmodern World*, Madison: University of Wisconsin Press, 1987.

59. McLaren, P. Schooling the postmodern body: critical pedagogy and the politics of enfleshment, *Journal of Education*, 1988, **170**, 3, 53–83.

60. Sarup, M. *An Introductory Guide to Poststructuralism and Postmodernism*, London: Harvester Wheatsheaf, 1994, p. 21.

61. hooks, b. Choosing the margin as a space of radical openness. In *Yearning: Race, Gender, and Cultural Politics*, Boston, MA: South End Press, 1990.

62. Bloch, cited in McLaren, *op. cit.*, p. 64.
63. Walker, 1993, *op. cit.* Walker, K. Confronting reality: nursing, science, and the micro-politics of representation, *Nursing Inquiry*, 1994, **1**, 46–56. Walker, K. Courting competency: nursing and the politics of performance in practice, *Nursing Inquiry*, 1995, **2**, 90–9. Walker, K. Crossing borders: bringing nursing practice, teaching and research together into the 21st century, *International Journal of Nursing Practice*, 1995, **1**, 1, 12–17.
64. See, for example, Lawler, J. *Behind the Screens: Nursing, Somatology and the Problem of the Body*, Melbourne: Churchill Livingstone, 1991. Holmes, C. Critical Theory and the Discourse of Nursing Ethics, Unpublished doctoral dissertation, Geelong: Deakin University. 1993. Parker, J.M. Bodies and boundaries in nursing: a postmodern and feminist analysis, paper delivered at the National Nursing Conference, Science, Reflectivity and Nursing Care: Exploring the Dialectic, 5–6 December 1991, Melbourne, Australia.
65. Bernstein, R. *Beyond Objectivism and Relativism*, Oxford: Basil Blackwell, 1983.
66. Foucault, cited in L.D. Kritzman (ed.) *Michel Foucault: Politics, Philosophy, Culture. Interviews and Other Writings, 1977–84*, A. Sheridan (trans.), London: Routledge, 1988, p. 154.
67. McLaren, P. Language, social structure and the production of subjectivity, *Critical Pedagogy Networker*, May/June 1988, Volume 1 and 2, 1–10.
68. Foucault, M. *Power/Knowledge: Selected Interviews and Other Writings 1972–1977*, C. Gordon (ed.), New York: Pantheon Books, 1980.
69. Flax, J. *Thinking Fragments: Psychoanalysis, Feminism and Postmodernism in the Contemporary West*, Berkeley: University of California Press, 1990, p. 6.
70. hooks, *op. cit.*, p. 153.
71. Lyotard, J. *The Postmodern Condition: A Report on Knowledge*, C. Bennington and B. Massunii (trans.), Minneapolis: University of Minnesota Press, 1984.
72. Britzman, D.P. *Practice Makes Practice: a Critical Study of Learning to Teach*, Albany: State University of New York Press, 1991, p. 6.
73. Spanos, cited in Lather, *op. cit.*,1991, p. 151.

CHAPTER FIVE

Postmodern research and reflective writing

*No man can think, write, or speak from his heart,
but that he must intend truth.*[1]

INTRODUCTION

Whereas Walker went 'all the way' and confronted the hegemony of empirical research and the written word head on, the general trend in nursing has been for accommodation and compromise, rather than for counter-hegemonic attacks. The usual way of adding credibility to the know-how embedded in narrativity has been to transform/translate the spoken narrative into written form, and it is perhaps no coincidence that the academic development of nursing during the 1990s was accompanied by a corresponding growth in reflective writing. In many ways, this reflective turn can be seen as part of a more general postmodern turn away from the legitimizing function of the metanarrative of scientific Method, and towards the multiplicity of individual little narratives. Emphasis is consequently shifted from research as the *discovery* and *verification* of external knowledge 'out there' in the world towards research as the *creation* of knowledge 'in here' by the researcher herself, in the act of writing it down; as Usher and Edwards pointed out, 'research is, above all, a textual practice of representation'.[2] Thus, whereas the modernist researcher would wish us to believe that the 'writing up' of the research is merely the final (and, in many ways, the least important) stage in a long and objective process of discovery, the postmodernist would argue that, by conforming to a particular narrowly defined style of scientific writing, the modernist researcher employs the write-up to perform two sleights of hand that disguise the true nature of research as a 'textual practice'. First, as Usher and Edwards continue:

> it is through a textual practice of writing that the creation, decontextualization and separation of the subject that researches from the 'object'

researched, a process considered essential to generating truthful representations and therefore to rigorous, 'scientific' research, is made possible.[3]

In other words, by conforming to a 'scientific' structure, the text assumes the objectivity supposedly guaranteed by the scientific method. Denzin refers to this as 'verisimilitude', which he described as 'the mask a text assumes as it convinces the reader it has conformed to the laws of its genre; in so doing, it has reproduced reality in accordance with those rules'.[4]

Second, the scientific researcher employs the write-up precisely to deny the textual nature of research. Thus:

> academic research texts are ostensibly about 'reality' but the reality in which they themselves are situated, from which they are produced and through which they can be read, falls out of view through decontextualisation.[5]

By being written in an 'objective' style (for example, in the third person), the very idea of research as a subjective text created by the researcher herself is implicitly denied; indeed, it is made unthinkable. Scientific research texts, then, 'can thus deny their own being as textual practices'.[6]

But if the creation of knowledge takes place at the time of writing, then, as Barthes claimed, the two are inseparable, and '"Research" is then the name which prudently, under the constraint of certain social conditions, we give to the activity of writing'.[7] This claim might, on first sight, seem a little strange: that we can create knowledge comparable to that produced by scientific research simply by sitting down and writing. However, it is only strange from the scientific perspective that truth and knowledge exist 'out there' in the world waiting to be discovered. If we adopt the postmodernist view that knowledge is a (largely linguistic) construct, and that the form that knowledge takes depends on the methods employed in its construction (and, indeed, on the language game played by the researcher), writing reflectively from our own experiences simply produces a different, but equally valid, kind of knowledge from that obtained from scientific research.

As I attempted to show earlier, knowledge and power cannot be separated. If we subscribe to this view that knowledge is validated and given credibility by those in power, the reason that scientific knowledge has a higher status than the knowledge produced by writing is not that it is somehow 'better quality' knowledge, nor even that it is more useful to practitioners, but instead that it is in the interest of those in power (in the case of nursing, mainly academics and researchers) to promote it as being of a higher status. As Foucault maintained, 'power produces reality, it produces domains of objects and rituals of truth'.[8] If the discipline were organized differently, if practitioners themselves were in control of their own profession (that is, in influential positions as journal editors, university professors and the administrators of research budgets), it is not difficult to imagine a situation in which reflective writing rather than the randomized controlled trial would be the 'gold standard' of knowledge generation.

Reflective writing, then, can be seen as a method of creating knowledge that has evolved in response to the conflicting demands of modernism and postmodernism. It is an attempt simultaneously to perpetuate the (postmodern) little narratives of the oral tradition of nursing practice and to conform to the (modernist) demands for a written, text-based academic discipline. However, while it has largely failed in its modernist bid for academic credibility,[9] reflective writing has not merely adapted the oral narrative form to a new medium, but has transcended it. Derrida, in particular, has noted that writing is not just a representation of the spoken word, but something more, such that 'the concept of writing exceeds and comprehends that of language'.[10] Thus, in a (postmodern) world in which 'there is nothing outside of the text',[11] writing is the perfect medium for the creation of knowledge. This theme is developed by Rolfe in the discussion that follows.

GARY ROLFE ON 'WRITING OURSELVES'

Rolfe begins from a point almost diametrically opposed to that of Walker, claiming that nurses should pay more rather than less attention to writing, since 'writing has intrinsic value as an academic activity and... is essential to our development as lecturers, researchers and nurses'.[12] He cites Jacques Derrida and Roland Barthes in an attempt to distinguish between writing and speech, and argues that when we write, we are doing something quite different from when we speak: writing is thought out and considered, whereas speech is immediate and impulsive. Unlike Walker in the previous chapter, Rolfe comes down firmly on the side of writing. On closer inspection, however, their positions are not as far apart as might be imagined; they both envisage the same ends, although their means of achieving those ends are rather different.

The key to the similarities between their two positions is that Rolfe is not simply arguing for writing, but for what he refers to as *writing*.[13] The difference is crucial: writing performs a number of functions, among which is accurate recording of thought and speech, the description of the world from the point of view of the writer, and analysis, 'the breaking down of knowledge in order to understand it'. *Writing*, on the other hand, goes further: 'in *writing*, we not only describe and come to understand our knowledge, but we can, in certain circumstances, construct it as we write'. *Writing* is therefore a creative act of synthesis, 'a way of constructing theory and knowledge in its own right', a method of doing research. This notion of *writing* as a research method is not to be confused with the modernist function of writing as the recording and dissemination of empirical research findings. The scientist writes in order to share her findings with others, usually after the research process is over. The *writer*, in contrast, *writes* to construct knowledge, and is herself unsure what will emerge until she begins to *write*.

Rolfe then goes on to argue that *writing* has much in common with Schön's notion of reflection-on-action, and he cites Max van Manen as suggesting that *writing* creates a specific state of mind in which reflection can take place, the so-called 'reflective cognitive stance'. For Rolfe, this has two important implications. First, the act of *writing* creates the mental state necessary for *writing*; and so, 'we create something new not by thinking about it, but by doing it; we write by writing'. It does not matter how much thinking time goes into the preparation for *writing*, the act of creation takes place as we *write*. Second, *writing* is therefore an end in itself, a creative act of knowledge generation. We do not *write* a book or a paper; we simply *write*. As Barthes pointed out, '*to write* is an intransitive verb',[14] and, as Rolfe adds, 'It is not what you write, but how... When we *write*, we are not merely creating ideas, we are creating ourselves; we *write* ourselves.'

This notion of writing ourselves is the key idea in Rolfe's paper, and it is in exploring this theme that his discussion takes the postmodern turn. Rolfe takes as his starting point the moment in 1968 when Barthes made his transition from structuralism to post-structuralism by announcing the death of the author. Echoing Lyotard's earlier remark that we live in a decentred universe, Barthes claimed that it is futile to attempt to decipher the original meaning placed in the text by the writer; instead, the job of the reader is to read her own meaning into it, to deconstruct and reconstruct, and ultimately to create something new. Rolfe merely takes the argument one step further by suggesting that this act of creation should involve not just a mental reconstruction in the head of the reader, but also a physical reconstruction on paper; that in order to create a new reading, we must create a new *writing*. Thus, as Rolfe points out, 'each individual reading of a text therefore has the potential to become a text itself'.

There is, of course, a difficulty with this notion, which Rolfe does not fully address – that of Derrida's problem of supplementarity, which was discussed in Chapter 2. Thus, if every reading of a text produces another text *ad infinitum*, we are in constant danger, as Spivak pointed out, of a 'fall into the abyss of deconstruction',[15] in which the original text is further decentred with every new reading. The danger, then, is that the authority of the original text is lost as it is pushed more and more into the margins by all the new writings emerging in response to it, writings that, from a modernist perspective, lack the authority of the original.

However, although Rolfe does not address the issue of supplementarity directly, he illustrates some of the difficulties associated with it through a literary example in the form of the short story 'The Library of Babel' by the Argentinean writer Jorge Luis Borges. Borges imagined a vast library of books containing every possible combination and permutation of letters; thus, somewhere in the library is a copy of every book that has ever been written, along with every book that it is possible to write. The mere thought is staggering. The library contains all that it is possible to express in words: all knowledge, all truth, including precise and detailed accounts of the past, present and future. Somewhere in the library is the book of my life, of your life, of all our lives.

This story makes a number of important points. First, it illustrates Rolfe's claim that writing is *qualitatively* different from speech. The spoken word cannot conceivably fulfill this function of cataloguing all that can be known; writing is achieved by combining letters to make intelligible words, opening up the possibility that something meaningful can arise from a random process (for example, the idea of an infinite number of monkeys producing the works of Shakespeare). The spoken word is, however, something quite different, and bears no direct relationship to the letters that form it. As Chesterton[16] observed:

> Man knows that there are in the soul tints more bewildering, more numberless, and more nameless than the colours of an autumn forest... Yet he seriously believes that these things can every one of them, in all their tones and semi-tones, in all their blends and unions, be accurately represented by an arbitrary system of grunts and squeals. He believes that an ordinary civilized stockbroker can really produce out of his own inside, noises which denote all the mysteries of memory and all the agonies of desire.

Second, it illustrates the link between language and knowledge, and, in particular, Wittgenstein's point that the language we use defines and constrains what it is possible to know. In a sense, then, language *creates* knowledge, and the limits of language also define the limits of knowledge.[17] Third, and most importantly, if everything that can be known is able to be expressed in words, then (written) language opens up the possibility of knowing everything. This idea is explored at length in Borges' story, in which the protagonist is at first optimistic and excited by the vertiginous thought that all knowledge is at his disposal; later his optimism turns to despair at the realization that not only all truth, but also all falsity is contained in the library; not only the true story of the world, but an almost limitless number of false stories as well. The possibility of knowing everything brings with it the realization that we can be sure of nothing. There might well be a real world, and there might well be 'true' knowledge about that real world; the problem is one of how we are to distinguish true knowledge from false knowledge.

This story prefigured by several decades the concerns of postmodernists, particularly the problem of the verification of knowledge: if (as Rolfe suggests) we are all to write, and some of what we write is contradictory, who is to act as the final authority? In a world without metanarratives, how do we decide which stories to accept and which to reject? For Rolfe, however, this is not a threat but a promise: the promise of liberation from the 'end' of nursing, that is, of a single metanarrative that prescribes where and how nursing should develop. The loss of certainty is therefore more than compensated by the gain of a creative profession, each practitioner 'with her own torch creating her own path through the darkness', writing her own script, inventing her own end.

Writing ourselves: creating knowledge in a postmodern world[18]

Gary Rolfe

WRITING AND SPEECH

Nursing, I have heard it said many times (but have rarely seen it written) is an oral tradition. When nurse education made the transition from the discourse of nursing to the discourse of higher education, it carried that tradition with it, and while there are growing numbers of nurse educationalists who are writing academic papers, they are still very much a minority. Several writers have attempted to address this problem in recent years. For example, Philip Burnard outlined the 'rules and skills of writing for publication',[19] noting that:

> The fact that the government runs a three-yearly exercise to monitor departmental productivity and the fact that part of that exercise involves an assessment of the department's publication means that nurse teachers not only have to teach: they must also publish.[20]

For Burnard, the UK government's Research Assessment Exercise (RAE) was a major justification for writing and publishing academic work, and writing was therefore validated as the means to the end of securing a good RAE score and earning money and prestige for the writer's university department.

While writing for the RAE is a commendable and necessary aim, and while I feel sure that Burnard recognizes other aims of writing, in this paper I intend to suggest a rather different set of reasons why all academics (and, indeed, all nurses) must write. I will argue that writing is not just a means to an end, whether that end be a paper, a text book or the RAE, but that it is also an end in itself; in short, that writing has intrinsic value as an academic activity and that it is essential to our development as lecturers, researchers and nurses. This paper, then, is not about *how* to write, which Burnard and others have already thoroughly and ably covered, but about *why* to write; in the face of claims that nursing is an oral tradition, it is a defence of writing, and more importantly (as we shall see), of *writing*.

But why, it might be asked, is writing so important? After all, there is a trend in nursing at the moment towards promoting and valuing tacit knowledge which cannot be expressed in words. Textbooks, it is claimed, can only take us so far; as experienced practitioners we move beyond written rules and procedures and rely on a form of intuition which Benner[21] referred to as expertise.

Or perhaps the value of writing is in preserving the spoken word, just as the student's written lecture notes attempt to preserve the spoken lecture, or published conference proceedings attempt to preserve the papers delivered at the conference. But these examples presuppose a correspondence between speech and text, that what is written acts merely as a permanent record of what has been said (either outwardly, or in the case of a journal paper, in the head of the writer).

This traditional view, in which 'writing is nothing but the representation of speech',[22] was referred to by the post-structuralist Jacques Derrida as 'phonocentrism'.[23] I wish to argue here, along with Derrida, that the act of speech and the act of writing are fundamentally different intellectual (and, of course, physical) actions. Roland Barthes, another post-structuralist, illustrated this difference when he wrote of the 'odour of speech'. Thus:

> As soon as one has finished speaking, there begins the dizzying turn of the image: one exalts or regrets what one has said, the way in which one said it, one *imagines oneself* (turns oneself over in image); speech is subject to remanence, it *smells*.[24]

On the other hand:

> Writing has no smell: produced (having accomplished its process of production), it *falls*, not like a bellows deflating but like a meteorite disappearing; it will *travel* far from my body, yet without being something detached and narcissistically retained like speech; its disappearance holds no disappointment; it passes, traverses, and that's all.[25]

When I speak, my words linger like a bad smell; I turn them over in my mind; I ask myself why I said X rather than Y; my words haunt and embarrass me long after their sound has faded away. As Barthes wrote: 'the time of speech exceeds the act of speech'.[26] In contrast, once I have written a text, once it is exactly how I want it, it is gone: it travels far from my body like a meteorite falling. The smell of the words I spoke at conferences five years ago still lingers; I can still remember how I felt at the moment of saying them. Papers I wrote five years ago are long forgotten; if I reread them it is as if they were written by someone else. As Virginia Woolf[27] pointed out, the self who writes is different from the self who later reads what is written. This objectification of the text is intensified when our writing is published, and:

> More so than long-hand writing, printed text is an object. We sense this in the greater ease with which we can take distance from our text once it has been converted into type-faced print.[28]

Why should this be? Why does speech smell in such a way? Barthes' answer was that speech slips from the tongue almost before we realise it has gone, and once gone, is irreversible: 'a word cannot be *retracted*, except precisely by saying that one retracts it'.[29] Text, however, is refined and perfected before it leaves the writer's protection, before it is made public. Thus, speech is the immediate and unmediated verbalization of thought, whereas a text is organized, justified, supported by reasoned argument. In speech, we jump around from point to point, we 'um' and 'er', we attack a point from several angles at once:

> The correcting and improving movement of speech is the wavering of a flow of words, a weave which wears itself out catching itself up, a chain of argumentative corrections which constitutes the favoured abode of the unconscious part of our discourse.[30]

In writing, however, we set out our thoughts in an orderly fashion, we are rational, the 'unconscious part of our discourse' is mediated and censored by the conscious. Thus, 'writing... taps the unconscious; it can make the implicit explicit, and therefore, open to analysis'.[31] Speech and text are not the same, and when we write we are not merely recording the (internally or externally) spoken word; we are doing something quite different.

WRITING AND *WRITING*

Writing as description

I do not, of course, wish to deny the descriptive function of writing; description and accurate recording are essential for the continuation of all but the most basic cultures, and progress, in the sense that it is usually understood in the west, is impossible without them. Thus, part of my reason as an educationalist for requiring students to write essays is concerned with the archival or descriptive function of writing; I wish to test their knowledge, or more accurately, their ability to describe an aspect of the world as they see it. This is the summative element of the essay. But if writing an essay was merely to assess what the student knows, then it would be a sterile and educationally suspect exercise. Writing, then, has certain other functions beyond the descriptive and the archival which are just as important, and I will now examine two of them in greater detail.

Writing as analysis

First, writing can be seen as a 'coming to understand', a way of checking out and making sense of what we think we know: 'writing teaches us what we know, and in what way we know what we know'.[32] This is writing as analysis; a breaking down of knowledge in order to understand it. In the process of writing an essay, the student comes to recognize and make sense of what she knows; knowledge is transformed into understanding as the student is forced to confront and rationalize an aspect of the world. This is the formative element of the essay: writing as a *means* to learning rather than merely as evidence of what has already been learnt.

Writing as synthesis

Second, and more importantly, writing is a creative act; in writing we not only describe and come to understand our knowledge, but we can, in certain circumstances, construct it as we write such that 'not until we had written this down did we quite know what we knew'.[33] This is writing as synthesis; the building up of something new from a variety of components. Many of us, I feel sure, have had this experience of not knowing quite what we are going to write until the very act of writing itself, and have been surprised by what emerged on the paper. The text you are now reading is primarily an attempt on my part to understand the nature of writing, to organize my thoughts on the subject. But it is also an effort to say something new, and what has emerged is not what I had originally intended to write; the ideas were formed during the act of writing itself. Thus, 'if we start by freely writing about the issue that concerns us, we will find ourselves expressing things not previously thought of'.[34]

This creative aspect of writing has been recognized by a number of social scientists as an important element of the research process. We write not only to record and make sense of the findings of research, but as a way of constructing theory and knowledge in its own right. For example:

It is not altogether fanciful to suggest that the act of 'interpretation' in interpretative sociology is as much an act of writing, of the organization of sociological texts, as it is a matter of cognitive processes of understanding.[35]

The process of knowledge generation in empirical research therefore continues after the data have been collected, and even after analysis has taken place. Schatzman and Strauss, for example, have argued that it continues right up until the researcher has finished writing up the findings:

> In preparing for any telling or writing, and in imagining the perspective of his specific audience, the researcher is apt to see his data in new ways: finding new analytic possibilities, or implications he has never before sensed. This process of late discovery is full of surprises, sometimes even major ones, which lead to serious reflection on what one has 'really' discovered. Thus, it is not simply a matter of the researcher writing down what is in his notes or head; writing or telling as activities exhibit their own properties *which provide conditions for discovery.*[36]

Barthes took this argument even further to suggest that the processes of research and writing are inseparable, and that 'research is then the name which prudently, under the constraint of certain social conditions, we give to the activity of writing'.[37] Writing can therefore be seen as a form of research in its own right, perhaps as the most basic and elementary form: it is an interrogation of the self which aims to uncover/create new knowledge and theory.

Van Manen argued not only that writing (what he called 'textual labor') was an essential part of the research act, but that it was equally important to reflection-on-action or what many nurses refer to as reflective practice. Reflection, he claimed, demands a certain form of consciousness, 'a consciousness that is created by the act of literacy: reading and writing'. Thus, 'writing is closely fused into the research activity and reflection itself'.[38]

This brings us back to the differences between speech and text discussed earlier. Text is not simply a written form of speech, but is something quite different which requires a different form of consciousness. Furthermore, as Van Manen pointed out above, it is a form of consciousness which is *created* by the act of writing; when we write, we are thinking in a different way. Van Manen continued by attempting to describe how writing creates this 'reflective cognitive stance':

> Writing fixes thought on paper. It externalizes what is in some sense internal; it distances us from our immediate lived involvements with the

things of our world. As we stare at the paper, and stare at what we have written, our objectified thinking stares back at us. Thus, writing creates the reflective cognitive stance that generally characterizes the theoretic attitude in the social sciences. The object of human science research is essentially a linguistic project: to make some aspect of our lived world, of our lived experience, reflectively understandable and intelligible.[39]

This suggestion that writing somehow creates the state of mind necessary to write, that our actions determine our cognitive state which in turn facilitates those very actions, is reminiscent of psychological behaviourism and the notion that, for example, we can lift a depression by 'pulling ourselves together' or 'pulling ourselves up by our own bootstraps' and acting as if we are not depressed. In fact, this notion of 'bootstrapping' can be seen not only in behavioural therapy but in early behaviourist descriptions of creativity and innovation:

> One natural question often raised is, how do we ever get new verbal creations such as a poem or a brilliant essay? The answer is that we get them by manipulating words, shifting them about until a new pattern is hit upon... How do you suppose Patou builds a new gown? Has he any 'picture in his mind' of what the gown is to look like when it is finished? He has not... He calls his model in, picks up a new piece of silk, throws it around her, he pulls it in here, he pulls it out there... He manipulates the material until it takes on the semblance of a dress... Not until the new creation aroused admiration and commendation, both his own and others, would manipulation be complete... The painter plies his trade in the same way, nor can the poet boast of any other method.[40]

We create something new not by thinking about it, but by doing it; we write by writing. But lest you dismiss this as mechanical and reductionist, here is C. Wright Mills, one of the most creative postwar sociologists, talking about what he called 'intellectual craftsmanship':

> As you rearrange [your writings], you often find that you are, as it were, loosening your imagination. Apparently this occurs by means of your attempt to combine various ideas and notes on different topics. It is a sort of logic of combination, and 'chance' sometimes plays a curiously large part in it.[41]

It is clear that these two very disparate writers, a behavioural psychologist and an anti-empirical sociologist, are saying much the same thing: that creative ideas occur at the time of the mechanical process of giving them shape. Our prior reading and experiences are the raw materials, but they are only turned into knowledge as we write.

The act of creation is therefore in the doing, and the creative state of mind, Van Manen's 'reflective cognitive stance' and Mills' 'loosening of the imagination', is engendered by the act of creation itself. Watson's dress designer manipulates the silk until he comes up with something original; Mills' intellectual craftsman (sic) rearranges her writing and combines various ideas until a new focus emerges, often largely by 'chance'. It is not chance, of course, or else we would all be famous dress designers and sociologists. But the point is that ideas often only crystallize during the physical act of writing them down: it is not enough merely to think or to speak; we must write.

The sociologist Howard Becker described the creative act of writing as a sustained process of rewriting draft after draft, and noted that creative writing is writing for discovery, not for presentation.[42] We are writing not for others but for ourselves, and at this level we might talk not merely of writing, but of *writing*. The writer writes to be read (usually by others), for presentation; the *writer writes* for the insights to be gained from the *writing*, for discovery. Writing is a means to an end; *writing* has intrinsic value and is an end in itself.

THE WRITER IS DEAD; LONG LIVE THE *WRITER*

In 1968, Roland Barthes made the transition from structuralism to post-structuralism by announcing the death of the author.[43] Because a text, once written, falls away from its author 'like a meteorite', so that the author no longer 'owns' the text, it therefore becomes public property and subject to 'readings' by whomsoever comes across it. It makes no sense, argued Barthes, to attempt to elicit the meaning which the author ascribed to the text, because there is no single 'objective' meaning. As Derrida claimed, we live in a 'decentred universe' without fixed points and absolutes.[44] Thus, it is the task of the reader (perhaps we should say, of the *reader*) to provide her own interpretation, her own reading. The reader therefore 'deconstructs' the text and thereby creates it anew. As Barthes pointed out, the death of the author entails the birth of the reader as the creative force in literature.

But we can take this argument a step further, particularly in relation to technical, scientific or academic texts (which Barthes did not consider). We might, as academics, deconstruct or read our own meaning into a scientific paper or a research report, but the creative act is really only complete when we *write* our reading, when we recreate (reconstruct) the text on paper. Ironically, then, the death of the writer leads us logically to the birth of the *writer*.

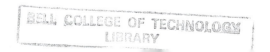

This notion of rewriting texts for ourselves is taken to the extreme in a (possibly tongue-in-cheek or 'ironic') short story by the Argentine writer Jorge Luis Borges. In this story, entitled Pierre Menard, Author of the Quixote, Borges imagines a twentieth-century writer named Pierre Menard who attempts to rewrite Cervantes' book *Don Quixote*.

> He did not want to compose another *Quixote* – which is easy – but *the Quixote itself*. Needless to say, he never contemplated a mechanical transcription of the original; he did not propose to copy it. His admirable intention was to produce a few pages which would coincide – word for word and line for line – with those of Miguel de Cervantes.[45]

Borges tells us that the first method Menard conceived was relatively simple(!): 'Know Spanish well, recover the Catholic faith, fight against the Moors or the Turk, forget the history of Europe between the years 1602 and 1918, *be* Miguel de Cervantes'.[46] However, this method was discarded in favour of the far more difficult task of 'to go on being Pierre Menard and reach the *Quixote* through the experiences of Pierre Menard'.[47] Menard finally managed to recreate, word for word, 'the ninth and thirty-eighth chapters of the first part of *Don Quixote* and a fragment of chapter twenty-two'.[48] Furthermore, 'although Cervantes's text and Menard's are verbally identical... the second is almost infinitely richer'.[49]

The story is written partly as a joke or parody. However, it forcibly makes the point that in order to really know a text, it is (almost) necessary to rewrite it from your own experience. Although Borges first published this story in the 1940s, well before Barthes announced the death of the author, it is interesting to note that in the preface to the 1981 edition, André Maurois wrote that:

> this subject, apparently absurd, in fact expresses a real idea: the *Quixote* that we read is not that of Cervantes, any more than our *Madame Bovary* is that of Flaubert. Each twentieth-century reader involuntarily rewrites in his own way the masterpieces of past centuries.[50]

I am merely (like Borges) taking this argument to its logical conclusion: that in order fully to engage with a text, any text, the reader must *literally* rewrite it, or rather, re*write* it. This should not entail a word-for-word mechanical transcription, nor an attempt to replicate the text *à la* Menard, but perhaps a writing *about* the text as a way of coming to understand it and, more importantly, of pushing its ideas further than did the original author. Each individual reading of a text therefore has the potential to become a text itself.

Taken to its extreme, this post-structuralist approach to writing brings us to postmodernism. Derrida famously proclaimed that 'there is nothing outside the text',[51] and the postmodernists interpreted this literally to mean that the world can be 'read' (interpreted) in the same way as a book. Another of Borges' short stories, again written in the 1950s but showing a stunning prescience, illustrates this attitude perfectly. In his story The Library of Babel, Borges imagined the world as an immense (and possibly infinite) library made entirely of hexagonal rooms:

> There are five shelves for each of the hexagon's walls; each shelf contains thirty-five books of uniform format; each book is of four hundred and ten pages; each page, of forty lines, each line, of some eighty letters which are black in colour. There are also letters on the spine of each book; these letters do not indicate or prefigure what the pages will say.[52]

Most of the books comprise a random jumble of letters, but occasionally a book would be found which contained one or more comprehensible words.

> One which my father saw in a hexagon on circuit fifteen ninety-four was made up of the letters MCV, perversely repeated from the first line to the last. Another (very much consulted in this area) is a mere labyrinth of letters, but the next-to-last page says *Oh time thy pyramids.*[53]

Over the years, the inhabitants of the Library (of the world) came to understand first that 'all the books... are made up of the same elements: the space, the period, the comma, the twenty-two letters of the alphabet';[54] and second that 'in the vast Library, there are no two identical books'.[55] This led to the inevitable conclusion that:

> the Library is total and that its shelves register all the possible combinations of the twenty-odd orthographical symbols (a number which, although extremely vast, is not infinite): in other words, *all that it is given to express, in all languages.* Everything: the minutely detailed history of the future, the archangels' autobiographies, the faithful catalogue of the Library, thousands and thousands of false catalogues, the demonstration of the fallacy of those catalogues, the demonstration of the fallacy of the true catalogue, the Gnostic gospel of Basilides, the commentary on that gospel, the true story of your death, the translation of every book in all languages, the interpolations of every book in all books.[56]

This is Derrida's claim that there is nothing outside the text taken to its literal(!) conclusion. The whole world is not only contained on the shelves of a library; the whole world *is* a library. It is, of course, quite impossible to imagine speech fulfilling the same role. Only text can generate all the possible permutations and combinations of letters to produce 'the translation of every book in all languages'[57] merely by chance (or in this story, by necessity).

The promise is therefore one of infinite knowledge; all is written, if only we search for long enough. Furthermore:

> It is verisimilar that these grave mysteries could be explained in words: if the language of the philosophers is not sufficient, the multiform Library will have produced the unprecedented language required, with its vocabularies and grammars.[58]

But the curse is one of uncertainty; how would we know the faithful catalogue of the Library among the 'thousands and thousands of false catalogues, the demonstration of the fallacy of those catalogues, the demonstration of the fallacy of the true catalogue'?[59] Thus, the Library (the world) is also a 'feverish Library whose chance volumes are constantly in danger of changing into others and affirm, negate and confuse everything like a delirious divinity'.[60] And ultimately, of course:

> An *n* number of possible languages use the same vocabulary; in some of them, the symbol *library* allows the correct definition *a ubiquitous and lasting system of hexagonal galleries*, but *library* is *bread* or *pyramid* or anything else, and these seven words which define it have another value. You who read me, are You sure of understanding my language?[61]

When we have access to everything, we can be certain of nothing. Furthermore, claimed Borges, the promise of truth and certainty is ultimately an illusion and the quest for it results in insanity.

Had it been written forty years later, Borges' story might have been interpreted (read) as a comment about the growth of the internet and the vast array of information to be found there (I recently heard a joke: it is said that a million monkeys randomly hitting the keys of a word processor would eventually produce something intelligible; the internet has shown this not to be the case). Nevertheless, it certainly prefigured the postmodern stance of an attitude of total scepticism, of 'incredulity toward metanarratives',[62] and in particular towards the 'enlightenment narrative, in which the hero of knowledge works toward a good ethico-political end – universal peace'.[63]

In this statement, Lyotard was challenging what Habermas had referred to as the 'incomplete project' of modernity which started with the Enlightenment and had as its (as yet unfulfilled) end the rationalization of human society.[64] But for Lyotard, history has no 'end', that is to say, no ultimate goal prescribed by a metanarrative. History is open-ended; there is no light at the end of the tunnel because there is no single tunnel and no single end, merely *writers*, each with her own torch creating her own path through the darkness. And perhaps the same is true of nursing: there is no metanarrative, whether it be science or humanism/holism, and no end; the vision of nurses marching side-by-side to the end of the tunnel of 'health', 'holistic care' or whatever is perhaps simply an illusion perpetrated by those with the power to define and censure nursing knowledge.

PULLING OURSELVES TOGETHER

But if this is the case, then we must all *write*, and not necessarily for publication but for ourselves. *Writing* defines who we are and what we think, it is our own personal torch to (en)light(en) the darkness. And nor does it matter what we write. Content is, in a sense, unimportant since writing is an end in itself: '*to write* is an intransitive verb', claimed Barthes,[65] a verb without an object, an end in itself. We do not *write* books or papers, we just *write*. It is not *what* you write, but *how*, as Borges' story about the *Quixote* demonstrated. When we *write*, we are not merely creating ideas, we are creating ourselves; we *write* ourselves.

But what exactly does it mean to *write* ourselves? We have seen that *writing* is a creative act of synthesis, of pulling together disparate elements to construct something new. We can think of the self as an aggregation of thoughts, knowledge, opinions, attitudes, ideas and other mental states (as Descartes famously wrote: 'I think, therefore I am'), and as Ornstein pointed out:

> the separate mental components have different priorities and are often at cross purposes, with each other and with life today, but they do exist and, more soberly, 'they' are us.[66]

Our *writing* therefore manifests our self (or, more accurately, our selves) on paper; it pulls together our disparate thoughts, attitudes and opinions and gives them a focus. To use the metaphor employed earlier, when we *write* we are 'pulling ourselves (our selves) together'.

This notion of *writing* as the synthesis or manifestation of self is succinctly illustrated in the Translator's Preface to Derrida's book *Of Grammatology*, where Spivak (the translator) briefly described Derrida's life and academic achievements, ending with a list of his published books. She concluded: 'Jacques Derrida is also this collection of texts'.[67] Roland Barthes made a similar point, claiming 'I am writing a text and I call it R.B.'[68] You are what you write.

To return to the claim I made at the start of this paper, that *writing* is essential to our development as nurses, lecturers and researchers, we can make a direct comparison between, for example, the act of *writing* and the act of teaching. Like *writing*, good teaching is also a form of synthesis, of pulling together knowledge and opinion from a variety of sources and offering it as a coherent package; a 'body' of knowledge. It is, of course, possible to teach solely from one or more books, but most experienced teachers offer their students a mix of 'book' knowledge and personal experience, knowledge and opinions, that is, something of themselves. Otherwise, we might just as well send our students off to read the books and all go home, reducing the function of universities as merely to award degrees (and, of course, there are some cynics who would claim that this is precisely the direction in which universities are heading). Thus, in order to teach, we must synthesize, and in order to synthesize, we must *write*. For example, in order to teach a class on, say, action research, I must first pull together what I know about the subject. This includes what I have read in books, heard at conferences, learnt from supervising students' dissertations, experienced from doing my own research projects, and so on.

These 'elements' of what I know are, in a way, the dismembered parts of my unique body of knowledge about action research. I carry them all in my memory, but it is impossible (at least for *my* brain) to consider them all at the same time. It is only when I write them down that I can pull them together into a coherent body of knowledge and come to recognize the totality of what I know about action research (we have all, I am sure, had the experience of trying to follow a complex argument from a verbal conference presentation: statements made five minutes previously are forgotten; we cannot go back and review them. Our brains can only hold so many concepts at one time).

But often the whole is greater than the sum of its parts. When I see these disparate elements all together in one place, on one piece of paper, I begin to make connections between them: as Watson described earlier, I shift my words about until a new pattern is hit upon; as Mills claimed, I 'loosen my imagination' by combining various ideas on different topics. And this often results in something new: a new angle, a new theory, a new 'reading' which has only come about because I have 'objectified' my subjective thoughts by writing them down. If my practice (whether of teaching, of nursing, or whatever) is to contain anything new, then I must *write*. I might submit my *writing* for publication, but that is not the reason why I *write*. I *write* in order to learn and I *write* in order to practise. As Becker said: 'this one is for discovery, not presentation'.[69]

NOTES

1. Blake, W. *All Religions Are One*, 1788.
2. Usher, R. and Edwards, R. *Postmodernism and Education*, London: Routledge, 1994, p. 149.
3. *Ibid.*, pp. 149–50.
4. Denzin, N.K. *Interpretive Ethnography: Ethnographic Practices for the 21st Century*, Thousand Oaks: Sage, 1997, p. 11.
5. Usher and Edwards, *op. cit.*, p. 150.
6. *Ibid.*, p. 150.
7. Barthes, R. (1971) Writers, intellectuals, teachers. In R. Barthes *Image Music Text*, London: Fontana, 1977, p. 198.
8. Foucault, M. *Discipline and Punish: The Birth of the Prison*, New York: Pantheon, 1977, p. 194.
9. This can be seen from the academic journals, which are stuffed full of research reports and methodology papers, with barely a reflective journal to be seen. Journal writing is still seen as a useful exercise for students, but the *contents* of the journal are not usually given credibility as knowledge.
10. Derrida, J. (1967) *Of Grammatology*, G.C. Spivak (trans.), Baltimore: John Hopkins University Press, 1974, p. 8.
11. *Ibid.*, p. 158.
12. All unreferenced quotations are from Rolfe's section in this chapter.
13. It has been pointed out that Rolfe's use of italics is itself a textual ploy to emphasize the differences between writing and speech, since the words 'writing' and '*writing*' can only be distinguished when written down. Closs, S.J. and Draper, P. Commentary, *Nurse Education Today*, 1998, **18**, 337–41.
14. Barthes, R. To write: an intransitive verb. In R. Macksey and E. Donato (eds) *The Language of Criticism and the Sciences of Man*, Baltimore: John Hopkins University Press, 1970, pp. 134–45.
15. Spivak, G.C. Translator's preface. In J. Derrida *Of Grammatology*, Baltimore: John Hopkins University Press, 1976, p. lxxvii.
16. Chesterton, G.K. *G.F. Watts*, London: Macmillan, 1904, p. 88.
17. That is not to say that the *world* is created by language, or even that it has no existence independent of language, but only (following Rorty) that *knowledge about the world* is a linguistic creation.

18. First published in *Nurse Education Today*, 1997, **17**, 442–8.
19. Burnard, P. Writing for publication: a guide for those who must, *Nurse Education Today*, 1995, **15**, 117–20.
20. *Ibid.*, p. 117.
21. Benner, P. *From Novice to Expert*, California: Addison-Wesley, 1984.
22. Rousseau, J.J. Fragment inédit d'un essai sur les langues. In *The Social Contract and Discourses*, G.D.H. Cole (trans.), London: Dent, 1913.
23. Derrida, *op. cit.*
24. Barthes, R. *Image Music Text*, London: Fontana, 1977, p. 204, original emphasis.
25. *Ibid.*, p. 204, original emphasis.
26. *Ibid.*, p. 204.
27. Woolf, V. *A Writer's Diary*, Bungay: Triad Granada, 1978.
28. Van Manen, M. *Researching Lived Experience*, New York: State University of New York Press, 1990, p. 129.
29. Barthes, *op. cit.*, p. 190.
30. *Ibid.*, p. 191.
31. Holly, M.L. Reflective writing and the spirit of inquiry, *Cambridge Journal of Education*, 1989, **19**, 1, 71–80.
32. Van Manen, *op. cit.*, p. 127.
33. *Ibid.*, p. 127.
34. Ferrucci, P. *What We May Be*, New York: St Martins Press, 1982, p. 75.
35. Hammersley, M. and Atkinson, P. *Ethnography: Principles in Practice*, London: Routledge, 1983, p. 209.
36. Schatzman, L. and Strauss, A. *Field Research: Strategies for a Natural Sociology*, Englewood Cliffs, NJ: Prentice Hall, 1973, p. 132, emphasis added.
37. Barthes, *op. cit.*, p. 198.
38. Van Manen, *op. cit.*, p. 125.
39. *Ibid.*, pp. 125–6.
40. Watson, J.B. *Behaviourism*, London: Kegan Paul, 1925, p. 198.
41. Mills, C.W. *The Sociological Imagination*, Harmondsworth: Penguin, 1959, p. 221.
42. Becker, H.S. *Writing for Social Scientists*, Chicago: University of Chicago Press, 1986.
43. Barthes, *op. cit.*, pp. 142–8.
44. Derrida, *op. cit.*
45. Borges, J.L. *Labyrinths*, Harmondsworth: Penguin, 1981, pp. 65–6.
46. *Ibid.*, p. 66.
47. *Ibid.*, p. 66.
48. *Ibid.*, p. 65.
49. *Ibid.*, p. 69.
50. Maurois, A. Preface. In Borges, *ibid.*, p. 12.
51. Derrida, *op. cit.*, p. 158.
52. Borges, *op. cit.*, p. 79.
53. *Ibid.*, p. 80.
54. *Ibid.*, p. 81.

55. *Ibid.*, p. 81.
56. *Ibid.*, pp. 81–2, emphasis added.
57. *Ibid.*, p. 82.
58. *Ibid.*, p. 82.
59. *Ibid.*, p. 81.
60. *Ibid.*, p. 84.
61. *Ibid.*, p. 85.
62. Lyotard, J.-F. *The Postmodern Condition: A Report on Knowledge*, Manchester: Manchester University Press, 1984, p. xxiv.
63. *Ibid.*, pp. xxiii-xxiv.
64. Habermas, J. Modernity – an incomplete project, *New German Critique*, 1981, **22**, 3–15.
65. Barthes, R. To write: an intransitive verb. In R. Macksey and E. Donato (eds) *The Language of Criticism and the Sciences of Man*, Baltimore: John Hopkins University Press, 1970.
66. Ornstein, R. *Multimind*, Boston, MA: Houghton Mifflin, 1987, p. 24.
67. Spivak, *op. cit.*, p. ix.
68. Barthes, 1977, *op. cit.*
69. Becker, *op. cit.*

CHAPTER SIX

Postmodern research and the 'new' science

To see a World in a Grain of Sand
and a Heaven in a Wild Flower,
Hold Infinity in the palm of your hand
And Eternity in an hour.[1]

INTRODUCTION

The radical break with the metanarrative of science described in the previous two chapters is not the only direction that postmodern thought has taken; it has also attempted to assimilate itself *within* the scientific discourse by redefining that discourse as a series of little narratives. As Lyotard pointed out, the metanarrative of science is beginning to be questioned not only by postmodernists, but also by scientists themselves, and, ironically, it has been the very success of science, particularly of physics, in probing ever deeper into the subatomic world that has prompted scientists to start to doubt the metanarrative of classical scientific method in favour of what Lyotard referred to as 'postmodern science'.[2] From this perspective, postmodernism does not lie in opposition to science; instead, science itself (and physics in particular) is beginning to uncover features of the natural world that appear distinctly postmodern, features that the classical scientific method is ill suited to dealing with. Thus, the eminent physicist Werner Heisenberg observed that:

> The violent reaction on the recent development of modern physics can only be understood when one realizes that here *the foundations of physics have started moving*; and that this motion has caused the feeling that the ground would be cut from science.[3]

Similarly, the physicist Niels Bohr wrote that 'the great extension of our experience in recent years... has shaken the foundation on which the customary interpretation of observation was based',[4] while

Einstein noted that 'it was as if the ground had been pulled out from under one, with no firm foundation to be seen anywhere, upon which one could have built'.[5]

This feeling that the very foundations of science were shifting, that the ground had been cut from beneath the feet of scientists, arose not just from the observation that, on a subatomic level, the world was a far stranger place than anyone had previously imagined, but also, far more profoundly, from the realization that many of the basic tenets that underpinned the metanarrative of scientific method were out of step with the emerging picture of what the world was really like. Most strikingly, the notion of objectivity, of the scientist standing back and remaining detached from what she was observing, completely broke down at the subatomic level. As the physicist John Wheeler noted:

> it destroys the concept of the world as 'sitting out there', with the observer safely separated from it by a 20 centimeter slab of plate glass. Even to observe so minuscule an object as an electron, he must shatter the glass. He must reach in... To describe what has happened, one has to cross out that old word 'observer' and put in its place the new word 'participator'.[6]

As Wheeler pointed out, even the mere act of observing a subatomic particle changes the way it behaves, so at the subatomic level, the distinction between observer and observed, between researcher and subject, on which the classical model of science is founded, breaks down. Thus, for Heisenberg, 'natural science does not simply describe and explain nature; it is part of the interplay between nature and ourselves'.[7] It is impossible to step outside the situation and view it objectively, since 'what we observe is not nature itself, but nature exposed to our method of questioning'.[8] The researcher is intimately connected with the subject of her research, not just on a figurative or metaphorical level, but physically. As Bohr maintained, 'isolated material particles are abstractions, their properties being definable and observable only through their interaction with other systems',[9] and as David Bohm added, 'one is led to a new notion of *unbroken wholeness* which denies the classical idea of analysability of the world into separately and independently existing parts'.[10] The claim by some nurses for a research methodology that takes into account the holistic nature of the person (and, indeed, of the entire physical world) is thus supported not just by a few cranky qualitative researchers and 'new age' philosophers, but also by some very eminent physicists.

This rejection of the possibility of an objective viewpoint is only one element of a more general questioning of the fundamental tenets of science. For Lyotard, the metanarrative of classical science rests on the notion that the physical universe behaves like a closed and highly stable system in which predictions about the future can be made from (the possibility of) a perfect knowledge of the present. Lyotard offered two reasons why this notion no longer applies in the subatomic world of the 'new physics', reasons that are not limited by external factors such as cost, 'but by the very nature of matter'.[11] First, he claimed, it is impossible fully to define or describe the initial state of a system, since such an undertaking 'would require an expenditure of energy at least equivalent to that consumed by the system to be defined'.[12] This objection, however, applies not only at the subatomic level. Lyotard cited the work of Benoit Mandelbrot on fractal geometry (which was later to become the mathematical foundation of chaos theory) as evidence that a complete description of a system is impossible, particularly:

> if, for example, we wish to make a precise measurement of the coast of Brittany, the crater-filled surface of the moon, the distribution of stellar matter, the frequency of bursts of interference during a telephone call, turbulence in general, the shape of clouds. In short, the majority of objects whose outlines and distributions have not undergone regularization at the hands of man.[13]

Fractal geometry suggests that 'the degree of [ir]regularity remains constant over different scales',[14] so that however closely we examine an object, it never displays a measurable smoothness. Thus, the coast of Brittany, as viewed from a satellite, displays a certain degree of irregularity containing some smooth and some rough, irregular parts. If we zoom in on a seemingly smooth portion of the coastline, that too, on closer inspection, displays the same unmeasurable irregularity. If we then zoom in even further, the smooth curves that appear to make up the overall irregular pattern always reveal an irregularity of their own. If we wish to measure the coastline, the result will depend on the degree of magnification that we use. If we attempt to measure the coastline of Brittany from a satellite picture of the world, the resulting length will be less than if we were to measure it from a more detailed picture of Europe, since extra curves will appear that were not visible in the smaller image. The more we zoom in, the more twists and turns become apparent, so the bigger the measurement becomes. Thus, there would be 'a kind of relativity in which the position of the observer, near or far, on the beach or in a satellite, affected the measurement'.[15] Furthermore, we will never attain a level of magnification at which a 'perfect' measurement is possible.[16] For Lyotard, this suggests that accurate measurements, even at the macro, everyday level, cannot be made. Like the subatomic physicist, the geographer is not measuring 'nature itself', but 'nature exposed to our method of questioning', and nature will yield different answers depending on whether our method of questioning involves taking measurements from a satellite picture or standing on the beach with a tape measure. There is no 'right' answer to the question, 'How long is the coast of Brittany?'

Even supposing, however, that we are able to obtain a precise and accurate measurement of the initial state of a system, Lyotard argued that it is still not possible to predict its future state. On the subatomic level, this can be seen, for example, in Heisenberg's uncertainty principle, 'which states that everything we can measure is subject to truly random fluctuations',[17] and thus 'an element of genuine unpredictability is... injected into nature',[18] while on a macro level, chaos theory tells us that a small initial fluctuation in the input to a system can cause an enormous change in its output. This so-called 'butterfly effect', coined from the title of a paper by its originator Edward Lorenz,[19] is concerned with 'the way that predictive errors evolve with time'.[20] Furthermore, 'any input error multiplies itself at an escalating rate as a function of prediction time, so that before long it engulfs the calculation, and all predictive power is lost'.[21] To all intents and purposes, then, most complex systems (and most systems in nature *are* complex) behave in random ways that cannot be predicted by even the largest and fastest computers. Furthermore, however large and fast the computer might be, it could *never* predict their behaviour, since it would be dealing with true randomness rather than merely with enormous complexity.

The case for a postmodern science therefore rests on the argument that classical science evolved to explain and predict a Newtonian mechanistic universe in which the researcher could stand outside the system she was observing, could (at least in theory) make precise measurements of the state of the system in the present, and could make accurate predictions about its state at any given time in the future. However, scientists now believe that the universe does not behave in such a way, and that Newtonian physics is only an approximation that breaks down on the micro, subatomic level, and even on the everyday macro level when complex systems are involved. Thus, for Lyotard, scientific Method as a metanarrative, as an overarching set of rules that can underwrite the findings of research in all situations and at all times, is no longer tenable; science has lost its universal authority. Instead of searching for universal truths, science is involved in a search for counter-examples, for paradox – what Lyotard referred to as the practice of 'paralogy'.[22] Thus, in place of a metanarrative, he proposed a 'temporary contract'[23] among scientists, in which 'any consensus on the rules defining a game [in this case, the game of science] and the "moves" playable within it *must* be local, in other words, agreed on by its present players and subject to eventual cancellation'.[24] We have, then, a new 'postmodern' science, with new, local and temporary rules, in which scientists and researchers are free to experiment outside the usual constraints of what was previously considered to be 'good science'. Postmodernism is not set up in opposition to science; instead, science has become postmodern.[25]

JOELLEN GOETZ KOERNER ON POSTMODERN SCIENCE

In the following discussion, Koerner explores some of the ways in which this postmodern science could be applied to nursing, and, in particular, to nursing management and administration. She notes that, historically, nursing has grown out of a modernist, quantitative Newtonian paradigm of science, although it has recently seen a shift to more qualitative methodologies, albeit still within a broadly modernist world-view. This paradigm tends to treat the universe as a machine, 'ticking along with clockwork precision',[26] and offers the promise of 'predictability, stability and control' via the elements of the world being broken down and analysed in smaller and smaller parts. Eventually, however, we reach what Koerner refers to as the 'quantum field', at which point 'Heisenberg's uncertainty principle replaced predictability, while chaos theory showed that most systems are nonlinear, dynamic, and ever-changing'.

It is perhaps worth pausing at this point to examine some of Koerner's terminology, particularly in view of Sokal and Bricmont's devastating critique of the misapplication of scientific concepts by postmodernist and post-structuralist writers. Koerner appears to be using the term 'quantum' fairly loosely as the 'general term for the indivisible unit of any form of physical energy',[27] in much the same way as the Ancient Greek philosopher Democritus employed the word 'atom', that is, as being the smallest possible particle that cannot be further subdivided. The term 'quantum field' is thus employed in the sense of activity at the (irreducible) quantum level.

Koerner's use of the term 'nonlinear' in relation to chaos theory is rather more problematic; as Sokal and Bricmont stated, 'it is frequently claimed that so-called postmodern science – and particularly chaos theory – justifies and supports this new "nonlinear thought". This assertion, however, rests simply on a confusion between the three meanings of the word "linear".'[28] First, the word is used to differentiate between linear and non-linear equations, but as Sokal and Bricmont pointed out, 'Newton's "linear thought" uses equations which are perfectly *nonlinear*', whereas 'the fundamental equation of quantum mechanics – Schrödinger's equation – is absolutely *linear*'.[29] Second, the word is used to describe 'linear order', as, for example, in the set of real numbers. However, Sokal and Bricmont claimed that there is also a third meaning, that of 'linear thought', which is employed by postmodernists to describe 'the logical and rationalist thought of the Enlightenment and of so-called "classical" science'.[30]

The problem, as Sokal and Bricmont saw it, is that this third meaning is loosely related to the second, the mathematical concept of linear order, yet is too often employed in relation to the first. However, while they took great pains to show that there is no absolute relationship between chaos and non-linearity, they ended up by tying themselves in logical knots. Thus, they pointed out that 'contrary to what people often think, a nonlinear system is not necessarily chaotic', but conceded that 'for chaos to occur, it is necessary that the equation be nonlinear and... not explicitly solvable'.[31] In other words, all chaotic systems are non-linear, but *not* all non-linear systems are necessarily chaotic. This does not, of course, refute the point that writers such as Lyotard were making, nor does it necessarily contradict Koerner's association of chaos theory with non-linearity. Ultimately, while Sokal and Bricmont's objection is valid against writers who specifically invoke non-linear *equations* in relation to chaos theory,[32] they added the disclaimer that 'we are *not* criticizing... authors for employing the word "linear" in their own sense: mathematics has no monopoly on the word'.[33] We must be careful, then, when reading Koerner, not to interpret her use of such terms as 'non-linear' in their strict mathematical sense.

Returning to Koerner's argument that, on the quantum level, the world is unpredictable and ever changing, she claims that this has led to an 'existential crisis' that requires a new way of looking at ourselves and our place in the universe, a new paradigm. Thus, 'the emergence of discoveries leading to the quantum field phenomena challenges humanity to look at the findings of the modern era with new eyes, lending new and broadening interpretation... to it'. Unfortunately, however, the social sciences in general, and the health sciences in particular, have been slow to respond; they continue to be locked into the reductionist 'classical science' model of analysing the world into smaller and smaller parts without paying due regard to the profound implications of quantum physics. So, for example, 'by breaking things down to their smallest parts we have become so narrowly focused and short-sighted that we are destroying our ecology and our broader economic systems... we have lost sight of community... [and] we have dehumanized work and the people we serve'.

Koerner is, however, optimistic that nursing science is beginning to take the postmodern turn. Unlike Walker in Chapter Four, who saw 'the North American icons of nursing's intellectual work' (although he did not name names) as attempting to assimilate nursing into the discourse of classical science, Koerner argues that writers such as Martha Rogers, Margaret Newman and Rosemary Rizzo Parse have all incorporated aspects of postmodernism into their models and theories. However, Koerner's main focus is not nurse theorists but nurse administrators, and she devotes the remainder of her chapter to an exploration of 'new ways to create systems and processes that are meaningful for all involved'.

Koerner begins by noting that the ordering process for both individuals and organizations in a mechanistic, Newtonian, systems-based model is based around 'a series of inputs that [are] processed in well-defined, discrete ways to obtain a desired output', that is, on a view of the whole being equivalent to the sum of its parts, which can be broken down, manipulated and rebuilt. In contrast, she argues, the postmodern world-view sees systems as organic, living entities that function according to four principles, and that must be studied holistically.

The first principle that governs a system is 'self-organization', by which Koerner means that systems should be viewed as a series of interdependent, interrelated organisms, bound together by a 'morphic field'[34] that 'articulates the vision and essence of a shared work'. Thus, Koerner claims that systems function best when they are subject to 'guiding processes' rather than 'rigid scripts', and she offers 'caring inquiry' and 'caring practice' as two such guiding processes for nursing.

The second principle is 'self-regulation', which 'combines competencies and evaluation to promote high levels of stability'. Thus, systems require clearly articulated competences for internal stability, and well-defined individual boundaries, which, continuing the living organism analogy, Koerner likens to a healthy cell membrane. This clearly articulated set of competences 'makes individuals and organizations less vulnerable to environmental fluctuations; it develops proactive autonomy that makes it unnecessary to always be reactive'. To stay viable, however, all living things must maintain a state of non-equilibrium, 'a fluctuating pattern of exchange with the world that promotes growth and renewal'. Thus, systems also constantly need to evaluate their internal and external relationships, which is attained through feedback loops for stability, and feedforward loops for creativity.

The third principle is that of 'self-generation', 'the processes used by organizations to manage information in life-giving ways'. Relating back to her earlier claims about uncertainty in postmodern science, Koerner suggests here that we need to relate to information in new ways: we must look for disturbance and fluctuations rather than stable trends (for example, in staffing patterns); we must look for paradox instead of tidy explanations (this, of course, is Lyotard's call for paralogy in science); and we must move beyond the obvious and seek the subtle (for example, in recognizing the value of clinical intuition).

The final principle is 'self-renewal', 'the creative capacity of the healthy organism'. For Koerner, this refers to the adaptive capacity to respond to others in creative and collaborative ways, the issue being 'not control, but dynamic connectedness'. Echoing the words of physicist John Wheeler, quoted above, Koerner claims that 'we live in a participative universe' in which 'we do not create reality, but are essential to its forthcoming'. This allows her to arrive at essentially the same conclusion as Rolfe in his chapter on writing, that 'action should precede planning, because only through action and implementation do we create the reality; we create it with our strong intentions'.

By any account, to advocate improvisation, experimentation, paradox, intuition and unplanned action, while claiming that 'the old prescriptive and safe ways of carrying out a prescribed set of tasks are the quickest way for any discipline to disqualify itself for the new reality', is a rather radical stance for a health services manager to take. In place of the 'old prescriptive and safe ways', Koerner wishes to see 'improvisational nursing', which 'calls us to develop a high level of self–other awareness; sharp sensing of intuition, feelings and imagination; a strong capacity for reflection in the moment; and, most of all, a this-AND-that versus this-OR-that mentality'.

However, this call for a new approach is based firmly on the belief that, although it might (in Sokal and Bricmont's words) be 'new age', it is nevertheless science. Koerner therefore ends with a call for a broadening out of scientific research to include multiple paradigms from a wide range of research traditions, and with a broad social agenda. Thus, 'We must start asking new questions: How is my practice affecting the community and the larger ecology? How are my thoughts impacting the mental ecology of the planet? How are my emotions affecting the emotional ecology of the planet? We must move from thinking *about nursing* to begin thinking *as nursing*, becoming deeply connected to life on every level of existence.' If, as Lyotard maintained, the atrocities of Auschwitz represent 'the tragic "incompletion" of modernity',[35] it is only fitting that the new project of postmodern science be founded on a broader ethical basis. By securing this global ethic to a scientific rationale, Koerner has attempted to do what the Enlightenment narrative allegedly failed to do: to produce a 'new Enlightenment' based on a new faith in a new science. Whether such a return to the promise of an emancipatory science merits the term 'postmodern' is something that will be explored in the following chapter.

Imagining the future for nursing administration and systems research[36]

JoEllen Goetz Koerner

INTRODUCTION

The art and science of nursing formulate the foundation for reflective professional practice. A reflective practitioner is one who demonstrates praxis – a theory-based practice. This professional mediates between his or her nursing practice and the universe of scholarly, scientific, academic discourse. Their practice is seen as part of a larger enterprise of knowledge generation and critical reflection. The reflective practitioner masters multiple techniques for formulation and production of scholarly knowledge as well as for testing, applying, or extending existing knowledge within the science of nursing. Such an awareness of the nature of knowledge as well as its limits are the hallmark of a mature practitioner who is personally, ethically, and professionally responsible. Nursing philosopher Kritek[37] observed that the nursing profession has had a unique journey toward science-based practice. Nursing began scholarly development by doing research, applying theories and methods from other disciplines. We then began to formulate theories, and now are starting to articulate a philosophy, while the reverse process occurred in most other fields. Historically, nursing practice and its research efforts have been deeply based in the quantitative, classic (modern) paradigm, largely focused on clinical aspects of client care. As nursing education moved into the academic setting, the studies were broadened to include nursing students, faculty, and the teaching–learning interface.

Within the past 10 years the research landscape shifted as a postmodern world-view emerged, bringing with it qualitative methods of inquiry. Simultaneously, nursing practice moved into a broader arena, with more practitioners involved in managing and influencing aggregate groups and systems, as in nursing administrative practice and case management practice. In the midst of this chaos, the nursing discipline is challenged to articulate and demonstrate its 'essence', its unique contribution to the health care field. Crafting a credible and defining research agenda within this diverse context requires nursing to redefine reality, reimagining its accountabilities and possibilities while acknowledging the perils of this scholarly path toward science-based practice.

PARADIGMS AND THE SCIENCE OF NURSING

Scientific principles established by Newton, combined with philosophical precepts uttered by Socrates, have formulated the foundation for the modern, science-based world-view that defines our present reality. This seventeenth-century linear model has formed and guided our observations, actions, and deliberation for more than 300 years (Figure 6.1).

Science	Philosophy
Physical sciences	Social sciences
Parts	Thoughts
To know	To understand
What is reality?	Who am I?
Microscopic view of health	Individualistic view of health
Germ theory	Behavioural theory

Figure 6.1   Modern world-view

The modern paradigm has several striking features that have deeply informed our sense of 'what is real'. Newton saw the world as a giant machine, ticking along with clockwork precision. This linear thinking model, based on the notion of predictability, stability, and control, was an honest attempt by scientists to 'know' and 'understand' how the universe is constructed and how it operates. Through the development of tools and models, modern science (nursing practice) evolved. Discovery occurred as elements were broken into small and smaller parts until we reached the quantum field. Heisenberg's uncertainty principle replaced predictability, while chaos theory showed that most systems are non-linear, dynamic, and ever changing.[38] These new findings have challenged all classic assumptions, creating the existential crisis and paradigm shift we are experiencing today.

However, discoveries from the classic era fostered the birth of a host of theories that describe the physical phenomena of the universe, including the phenomenon of health. Germ theory, one such model, became the foundation for early medical and nursing practice. Health was viewed as an absence of disease, and all activities were focused on the eradication of disease. Biological and chemical warfare were balanced with technologies used to diagnose and treat the invading agent, while care and comfort were provided to the individual engaged in this war. As science continues to unfold new agents and technology, we find variations to this theme in some professional practice models, although the basic premises remain.

Simultaneously, as the physical sciences were being probed, a companion activity was occurring in the philosophical realm; the search for 'who am I?' Society began as a tribal community with a collective mindset, consciousness, and set of cultural norms universally adopted to ensure survival. As the tribal unit gave way to state, national, and global awareness, humans' need to know themselves as unique individuals within the larger aggregate became a primary quest. The emergence of an alphabet, the printed word, and now satellite communications, have unleashed the exploding storehouse of knowledge to each individual rather than a few scholars who held 'truth' and interpreted it to the masses. Transglobal networks are expanding our connections, merging our awareness into a (quantum) field of knowing. As we acquire a broader personal consciousness, it changes our relationship to everything. As we understand self-in-relation more deeply, the arbitrarily drawn boundaries and distinctions seem irrelevant, or only partially correct, causing us to question relationships on all levels and our responsibilities within them.

As the philosophical/psychological dialectic expanded, health took on a broader definition. We began to see that stability, regularity, equilibrium, and 'the most fit' were hallmarks of health. Behavioural theories emerged in the sociological field and were reflected in the nursing world. Suddenly body, mind, and environment models emerged with adaptation interpretations. Nursing professionals, as experts in health, determined the best plan of care (based on nursing science) for the patient. Those not adhering to the master plan were labelled 'noncompliant', and manipulating interventions were introduced to get the patient back to centre.

At an organizational (hospital system) level, the modern worldview was also guiding the design of our care delivery systems and the way people performed within them. Classic physics holds that by identifying certain 'inputs' and putting them through carefully crafted 'throughputs' we can obtain desired 'outputs'. From a linear perspective, if something works well, more will work even better – establishing productivity measures. If you understand parts, you can understand the whole, so flow charts and discrete job descriptions neatly compartmentalize the work and the workers, only to be integrated by management thinking. The organization was viewed as a machine that needs structure and control to operate. Workers and their jobs are cogs in a wheel, precisely defined and monitored. Quality is assured by designing feedback loops to measure outcomes and keep them within preset benchmarks. Linear thinking poses that the future can be predicted from the past, that change is gradual and predictable. Thus, future forecasting was accomplished by looking at past trends.

Quantitative research methods and processes were well suited to examine and explain the phenomena being scrutinized in this era of history. But suddenly we stand in a crisis; we are at a watershed era in our history. The old ways seem to be only partial solutions to the situations we face. Dualistic, linear thinking does not address the complexity we face today. Categorical approaches such as either/or, good/bad, right/wrong, in/out, black/white, cannot respond fully to the paradoxical and dynamic phenomena in which our life experiences are nested. By breaking things down to their smallest parts we have become so narrowly focused and short-sighted that we are destroying our ecology and our broader economic systems. By becoming so autonomous and self-focused we have lost sight of community, with isolationism and violence destroying our social fabric. By viewing organizations as machines, workers as mere cogs, and patients as individuals to control, we have dehumanized work and the people we serve. Simultaneously, if we did not have the rich learning and discovery of the past 300 years, we would still be an unenlightened civilization. The propagation dance between science and philosophy has given birth to a new child: the quantum field. Society (nursing) is now called to use the foundational learning of our rich heritage and build enlarging life-giving models based on broader assumptions and applications as we approach the twenty-first century (see Figure 6.2).

We are at a major turning point, not merely of the human epic, but of the entire universe. To understand the meaning of an event, we must view it in terms of the bigger picture with a broader perspective. Anthropologists and cultural historians suggest that the largest possible context, the foundation for all meaning, is found in people's creation and rebirth story – their cosmology. Anthropologist Margaret

Quantum field
● Physical/social/human sciences
● Whole/parts relationships
● Make meaning – know and understand
● What purpose is all of life?
● Interdependent moral view
Modern world view
Health: quality of life in all dimensions – simultaneously

Figure 6.2   Postmodern world-view

Mead observed that every culture she ever encountered had a creation myth.[39] Each human being develops a unique set of stories that reveal 'truth' gathered from observation, intuition, and learning and the lived experience. This story set gives life its meaning and purpose, helps us know our place and destiny in the cosmos, and gives us a sense of right and wrong, good and bad. Our present cosmology based on classic physics principles offers an incomplete explanation for our lived experience. Gregory Bateson commented, 'The major problems in the world are the result of the differences between the way nature works and the way people think.'[40] Today we are experiencing a shift in perspective and identity, we are rewriting our cosmology story on every level of human existence.

Albert Einstein saw the emergence of our new reality later in his illustrious career. He remarked that

> science without religion is lame. Religion without science is blind. The unleashed power of the atom has changed everything except our way of thinking. Thus we are drifting toward a catastrophe beyond comparison. We shall require a substantially new manner of thinking if humanity is to survive.[41]

Discoveries in chaos theory, quantum physics, and mathematics are converging with discoveries occurring in the social, religious, and psychological arenas, bringing us to a new definition of reality and being. The space programme also gives us another physical perspective of reality and our place in the larger universe. Astronaut Frank White observed:

With all the arguments, pro and con, for going to the moon, no one suggested that we should do it to look at Earth. But that may in fact have been the most important reason of all. The clear message of seeing ourselves from space is that Earth is a whole system and humanity one of its many interdependent species. A regard for all of life as sacred becomes a practical as well as moral position when we see the critical role that all life plays in maintaining the system... If the next step in human evolution is to build a planetary civilization, then what is most needed is the ability to see and deal with problems and opportunities on a planetary level. It is also the ability not only to observe, but to truly communicate with the planet as a whole.[42]

The emergence of discoveries leading to the quantum field phenomena challenges humanity to look at the findings of the modern era with new eyes, lending new and broadening interpretation and application to it. We must place phenomena in a context illuminated with findings from the physical, social, and human sciences. We are called to consider whole–part relationships when making decisions, seeing short- as well as long-term implications for self, society, and the ecology. It is no longer sufficient to know and understand. We must move from 'what' and 'why' questions to the 'so what' inquiry that will bring us face to face with issues surrounding the meaning and purpose of all of life. We must move from an independent, self-focused decisioning process to one based on justice and goodness. Heffeman defines a thing as right when it tends to preserve the characteristic diversity and stability of the system. Thus, nursing is called to a higher level of discernment as health is defined as quality of life in all dimensions, simultaneously – as defined by the person.

Philosophical tenets of nursing have been articulated by Kritek.[43] Assumptions that guide postmodern practice (and our research agenda) include:

- *Health care* is a moral good; transacted by limited, imperfect, less than moral humans; ambiguous, at once noble and genuine, avaricious and cruel.
- *Evolution* occurs in time and space, future time and space, and is emergent from present time and space altered.
- *Health care providers* work within the parameters in the moment and place, with the profound limits of human nature.
- *Creativity* crafts new relations by crafting new relationships among a set of givens, and crafts new realities by bringing new focus into a given field of action, crafts new knowledge by bringing new knowing into a given field of attention.

Dr. Kritek states that postmodern philosophy dictates that all under-standing is rooted, contextual, and historic. When we critique our thought patterns through self-reflection, we discover the prejudice of the historic, rooted, and contextual. We must embrace what is happening in the moment, knowing that only love and fear exist. Foundational thought is both unnecessary and undesirable. We encounter 'experiences of truth' in the moment. In dialogue we discover the other's experience of truth. The goal of philosophy is to continue a conversation, not discover the truth; truth is an ongoing disclosure in the moment – each moment is truth. By framing the phenomenon in theory, we can discern its meaning.

Nursing theory based on nursing science is demonstrating an incor-poration of postmodern principles. Martha Rogers[44] defines the person as a unified and patterned energy field. Health is viewed as the patterning of the energy field with the environmental energy field. Nursing is the repatterning of person and environment to achieve the maximum health potential of the person. Newman[45] views the person as a centre of energy. Health is the expansion of consciousness, with the environment in continuous interaction and patterning with the person. Nursing facilitates repatterning of the patient to higher levels of consciousness by enhancing the awareness of individual choice patterns and possibilities available. Parse[46] sees the person as a patterned, open being, more than and different from the sum of its parts. Health is a continuously changing process of becoming in an environment that is in mutual and simultaneous interchange with the person. Nursing is an interactional process that facilitates the person in living the values of his or her choosing. Each of these theories is based on the simultaneity paradigm, placing the direction and choices for life back into the hands of the individual. There is also a deep recog-nition of the dynamic exchange with the environment, an environ-ment that has taken on new definition in the quantum world.

Nurse administrators, social policy makers, and others who have responsibility for capturing the phenomena of large groups over time, are seeking for new ways to create systems and processes that are meaningful for all involved. Further, they are looking for new tools and methods to measure and report phenomena occurring in the field. Guidelines for such work can be found in the quantum field.

The ordering process for individuals and organizations in a mecha-nistic, Newtonian system-based model was configured on a series of inputs that were processed in well-defined, discrete ways to obtain a desired output. Individual phenomena were controlled and quantita-tively measured in isolation with generalizations made for the whole.

The postmodern world calls for a very different ordering process. These new organic, living models are based on four major categories that must be studied differently if the phenomenon nested within is to be accurately identified; self-organization, self-regulation, self-generation, and self-renewal.[47]

Self-organization refers to the way a system is designed to hold itself together. Rather than being viewed as structured, isolated parts, new organizational systems are viewed as interdependent, interrelated organisms. Instead of these systems being held together by rigid organizational boundaries, the glue or morphic field that binds them is a self-organizing principle that articulates the vision and essence of a shared work. It is the purpose of the organization that unites and infuses each individual with meaning and commitment to a shared outcome. For nursing, the vision may be 'caring in the human health experience'.[48]

Guiding processes give direction rather than rigid scripts, allowing the individual practitioner freedom to co-create with the person, in the moment. Two guiding processes that may be studied to understand this organizing phenomenon are caring inquiry and caring practice.[49] Caring inquiry goes beyond the superficial to understanding what matters to the person from an insider's perspective.[50] Caring practice is doing for persons things that they cannot do for themselves at an ethical interface where the personal and professional experience of the nurse blends with the personal and health experience of the one seeking care. This is the unique gift that nursing makes to patients in the health care system. It is at this sacred interface that we witness incredible acts of the human spirit, and often both are changed in the experience. Although it is seldom recorded in the chart, and is not readily captured by numbers, this phenomenon reflects the essence of the profession. Such rich material can be captured through stories and phenomenologic modes of inquiry.

A second organizational ordering process is the notion of self-regulating. This self-referencing process combines competencies and evaluation to promote high levels of stability.[51] The foundation for identity and excellence in performance is a set of well-defined competencies. As nursing and science continue to evolve in complexity and density, it is essential that we differentiate our work in ways that increase the performance for all nurses, to better meet the evolving health care needs of society.[52] Clearly articulated competencies lead to internal stability and well-defined individual boundaries (like a healthy cell membrane), which then open to the outside (to maintain body integrity). This makes individuals and organizations less vulnerable to environmental fluctuations; it develops proactive autonomy that makes it unnecessary to always be reactive.

However, equilibrium is neither the goal nor the fate of living systems, simply because as open systems we partner with the environment. To stay viable we maintain a state of nonequilibrium, a fluctuating pattern of exchange with the world that promotes growth and renewal. Evaluation and reward structures, coupled with a dynamic continuous quality improvement process, maintain integrity of role contribution. Two guiding processes enhance evaluation; feedback and feedforward loops. The well-known feedback loop signals departure from a norm, identifying performance that must be redirected to preserve the system at its ideal level (for example, number of medication errors). Feedforward loops use the same information differently. These loops increase the discrepancy at the interface (amplifying it) so the disturbance can grow. Thus, areas of conflict and disagreement mark a rich interface between what was and what could be. The learning in this dissonant field holds a seed for new order, planted in the soil of intellectual capital. Here is a wonderful place to analyse phenomena through dialogue and probing, using multiple methods of inquiry such as logistic maps and phase plane analysis, to promote the creation of new order.[53]

Self-generation is the process used by organizations to manage information in life-giving ways. Like nourishment for a human body, information is creative energy. Information gives order to form; like DNA, it informs a system. In giving order, it promotes growth and defines what is alive, what lives. Communication generates order from the information. The greater our ability to process information, the greater is our level of awareness and the integrity of the people who share it. Organizational processes that house such activities include councils, task forces, and committees. The postmodern world requires us to relate to information in new ways. Along with averages, we must look for disturbances and fluctuations. Creating staffing patterns for a census of 350, when the organization experiences census swings from 210 to 420 each month, is not very meaningful to a staff called to stay home after working three extra shifts the previous pay period. We must look for paradox instead of tidy explanations. Whenever we discover a truth, we know that its opposite is also true. Independence is balanced with interdependence, change with stability, continuity with newness, autonomy with control. Rather than examining generalizations based on averages, by noting the paradox we are in a position to transcend them to a higher order. Finally, we must move beyond the obvious and seek the subtle. An exceptional nurse is the one who intuitively 'knows', when all clinical indicators are stable, that something is amiss with the patient. This same phenomenon holds true for administrators and researchers. We must value and use our intuition as much as our scientific reasoning to fully discern the situation under question.

Research around this phenomenon must ask different questions. We must abstract information from new connections between data and situations. We must seek insights from other disciplines, other places, going outside the nursing circles to get it. How can social policy research processes and outcomes inform our expanding research agenda? How can nursing administration create new productivity measures that transcend the outdated and meaningless full-time equivalent per adjusted occupied bed, and partner with the Health Care Financing Administration to alter benchmarks for the health care field? We must actively enlarge our circles of exchange and networking, moving into camps of dissent and lack of interest because we have something profound and pertinent to contribute to the evolving reality of health care delivery! Instead of waiting to be invited to the table, we must set a table of our own, and invite others in.

Finally, the evolving universe operates on the notion of self-renewal, the creative capacity of a healthy organism. This reflects the adaptive capacity to respond with spontaneously emerging structures through establishment of partnerships with the person, co-consulting relationships within nursing, and collaboration with other disciplines. The issue is not control, but dynamic connectedness. We live in a participative universe; we do not create reality, but are essential to its forthcoming. We evoke a potential that is already present. Acting should precede planning, because only through action and implementation do we create the reality; we create it with our strong intentions. The thing that gives power its positive or negative charge is the quality of the relationship. We must establish the relationship and then improvise the dance.

To explore nursing's contribution to health care we must examine our relationships and the improvisational activities that exist within them. The old prescriptive and safe ways of carrying out a prescribed set of tasks are the quickest way for any discipline to disqualify itself for the new reality. By combing through constantly changing information with others, available choices are noted and a response crafted. Openness and creativity that influence the evolution of systems and individuals also affect the environment. In a state of co-creation with partners, colleagues, and systems, all evolve simultaneously toward better fitness and health. Improvisational nursing calls us to develop a high level of self–other awareness; sharp sensing skills of intuition, feelings, and imagination; a strong capacity for reflection in the moment; and, most of all, a this-AND-that versus this-OR-that mentality.

DEVELOPING AN INCLUSIVE CULTURE OF INQUIRY

The doctoral programme at the Fielding Institute does not teach research. Its community of 800 students come from all over the world; thus they teach a course called Cultures of Inquiry. Such cultures are defined as general types of inquiry based on differing paradigms of knowledge: phenomenological, ethnographic, empirical-analytic, historical, or action research. To what extent is a culture regarded as scientific? The modern world held 'science' to mean the natural sciences with cool, detached observation, highly mathematical modelling, quantitative measurement, and prediction. This does not capture well what goes on in the human sciences. Humans, unlike atoms and molecules, think, live in a world where 'things' have symbolic rather than fixed meaning, and are capable of reflecting upon their world, often altering their behaviour as a result. Thus, in the postmodern world, 'science' has been enlarged to mean a commitment to using rational procedures and argument to bring about results that achieve broad agreement among a community of scholars.[54] While the goal of science is understanding, the nature of that understanding will vary according to the particular culture of inquiry. The ultimate goal of advanced education is creation of a scientific attitude, the reflective stance of a scholarly practitioner that entails a strong desire for understanding, an inquisitiveness, and a willingness to subject one's ideas and results to the critical scrutiny of others.

New methods of inquiry continue to be created, many of them nonexistent 25 years ago. Within the nursing literature, extensive debate has emerged concerning the methods and methodologies used within the field. A purist view that either a qualitative or quantitative approach is best, and one must never combine the two, is part of our current reality. In their provocative article calling for the coexistence of stories and numbers without compromise, Ford-Gilboe, Campbell, and Berman[55] make a compelling case for our confusion between method and methodology. According to feminist researcher Harding,[56] method refers to the particular procedures used to gather evidence in the course of research. Methodology, on the other hand, pertains to a theory of how research is carried out, the general principles about how to conduct research and how theory is applied. Ford-Gilboe and colleagues[57] pose the belief that more important than the selection of particular methods is the way in which these methods are used. Methods are not constrained by any particular paradigm; numbers and stories neither violate nor uphold paradigm assumptions. A broader perspective acknowledges the complementarity of quantitative and qualitative approaches to the development of nursing knowledge. The article clearly addresses issues of methodology and scientific rigour, and the final call is compelling. As nursing research moves into a postmodern era, multiple paradigms are acceptable for research. Rigid boundaries are limiting and often dictated by historic and political considerations rather than scientific or purely ontologic concerns. If nursing can focus on our shared concern – to produce good science that will improve the health and well-being of society – we will begin to recognize and value other paradigm insights in developing new and evolving discoveries on the forefront of knowledge creation.

The postmodern world-view is calling nursing to return to our roots, to reinvent ourselves in fresh, new yet old ways. Our origins began in the community, and it is to this sacred space that we are returning. Having spent the last 300 years nested within systems and cultures that were hierarchical and patriarchal, we learned many lessons that can now serve us well. Teilhard de Chardin[58] observed that what transcends, assimilates. We must rise above and out of that world, into one that redefines health as the well-being of the universe and everything in it. Nursing must become a proactive, reflective discipline, partnering with others to create a more humane society. We must move from defining ourselves and our patients in the singular, and create a larger social agenda. We must start asking new questions: How is my practice affecting the community and the larger ecology? How are my thoughts impacting the mental ecology of the planet? How are my emotions affecting the emotional ecology of the planet? We must move from thinking *about nursing* to begin thinking *as nursing*, becoming deeply connected to life on every level of existence.

How we perceive an individual human being, health, and nursing's work in our imagination literally makes a world of difference. Our true reality is that we are each an integral member of a world community. We are each part of a living community of diverse personalities bound together in an inseparable relationship in time and space. Everything is totally interdependent and interrelated. Thus, we have no existence apart from the earth. We are totally dependent upon the health of the ecology and the wider community of life for our own health. Our own destiny, the destiny of humanity, and the destiny of earth are identical. What we do to it, we do to ourselves. Let us reinfuse the light of nursing with an open consciousness that acknowledges the uniqueness of each individual, the rich diversity of the universe, and serve it with the flame of unconditional commitment to caring for its quality of life.

The day will come when, after mastering the wind, the waves, the tides and gravity, we shall harness for God the energies of love. And on that day, for the second time in the history of the world, humanity will have discovered fire.[59]

NOTES

1. Blake, W. *Auguries of Innocence*, 1803.
2. Lyotard, J.-F. (1979) *The Postmodern Condition: A Report on Knowledge*, Manchester: Manchester University Press, 1984.
3. Heisenberg, W. *Physics and Philosophy*, London: Allen & Unwin, 1963, p. 145, emphasis added.
4. Bohr, N. *Atomic Physics and the Description of Nature*, London: Cambridge University Press, 1934, p. 2.
5. Cited in P.A. Schipp (ed.) *Albert Einstein: Philosopher-Scientist*, Evanston, IL: Library of Living Philosophers, 1949, p. 45.
6. Wheeler, J.A. In J. Mehra (ed.) *The Physicist's Conception of Nature*, Dordrecht: D. Reidel, 1973, p. 244.
7. Heisenberg, *op. cit.*, p. 75.
8. *Ibid.*, p. 57.
9. Bohr, *op. cit.*, p. 57.
10. Bohm, D. and Hiley, B. On the intuitive understanding of nonlocality as implied by quantum theory, *Foundations of Physics*, 1975, **5**(1): 93–109, emphasis added.
11. Lyotard, *op. cit.*, p. 56.
12. *Ibid.*, p. 55.
13. *Ibid.*, p. 58.
14. Gleick, J. *Chaos: Making a New Science*, London: Cardinal, 1988, p. 98.
15. *Ibid.*, p. 162.
16. Mathematicians often illustrate this point by referring to fractal equations, which, when plotted on paper, produce such staggering shapes as the 'Mandelbrot set', which continues to reveal new complexities however much we zoom in on its details. As Gleick noted, 'In the mind's eye, a fractal is a way of seeing infinity': *Ibid.*, p. 98. You might wish to compare Gleick's statement with William Blake's poem at the start of the chapter.
17. Davies, P. (1991) cited in J. Carey (ed.) *The Faber Book of Science*, London: Faber and Faber, 1995, p. 499.
18. *Ibid.*, p. 499.
19. Lorenz, E. Predictability: Does the Flap of a Butterfly's Wings in Brazil set off a Tornado in Texas?, address to the annual meeting of the American Association for the Advancement of Science, Washington, 1979.
20. Davies, *op. cit.*, p. 499.
21. *Ibid.*, p. 500.
22. Lyotard, *op. cit.*, pp. 60–1.

23. *Ibid.*, p. 66.
24. *Ibid.*, p. 66.
25. Although some scientists might claim that, at this point, the language game being played is no longer that of science. As Gleick noted, 'where chaos begins, classical science stops'. *Op. cit.*, p. 3.
26. All unreferenced quotations are from Koerner's section in this chapter.
27. Walker, P.M.B. *Chambers Science and Technology Dictionary*, Edinburgh: Chambers, 1991, p. 730.
28. Sokal, A. and Bricmont, J. *Intellectual Impostures*, London: Profile Books, 1998, pp. 133–4.
29. *Ibid.*, p. 134–5, original emphasis.
30. *Ibid.*, p. 133.
31. *Ibid.*, p. 135.
32. In this respect, Sokal and Bricmont (*ibid.*, p. 134) pointed the finger specifically at Harriett Hawkins, Steven Best and Robert Markley.
33. *Ibid.*, p. 134.
34. The term 'morphic field' is probably a reference to the work of the anthropologist Gregory Bateson (whom she cites elsewhere), who was concerned with the processes by which living things organized their own growth, and also to René Thom's writing on morphogenesis, which Lyotard referred to in relation to postmodern science. It might also refer to Rupert Sheldrake's 'morphogenetic fields', which 'can be regarded as analogous to the known fields of physics in that they are capable of ordering physical changes, even though they themselves cannot be observed directly': Sheldrake, R. *A New Science of Life*, London: Paladin, 1981, p. 72. Koerner might not wish to be too closely associated with this latter concept, however, which Sokal and Bricmont (*op. cit.*, p. 244) disparagingly referred to as a 'new age fantasy'.
35. Lyotard, J.-P. *The Postmodern Explained to Children*, London: Turnaround, 1992, p. 30.
36. First published in *Nursing Administration Quarterly*, 1996, **20**, 4, 1–11.
37. Kritek, P. Negotiating at the Uneven Table, paper presented at Center for Nursing Leadership, Hill-Rom Farm, Batesville, Indiana, 1995.
38. Briggs, J. and Peat, D. *Turbulent Mirror: An Illustrated Guide to Chaos Theory and the Science of Wholeness*, New York: Harper & Row, 1989.
39. Dowd, M. *Earthspirit: A Handbook for Nurturing an Ecological Christianity*, Mystic, CO: Twenty Third Publications, 1991.
40. Bateson, G. *Steps to an Ecology of Mind*, New York: Ballantine, 1972, p. 114.
41. Dowd, *op. cit.*, p. 7.
42. *Ibid.*, p. 100.
43. Kritek, *op. cit.*
44. Rogers, M.E. Science of unitary human beings. In V.M. Malinski (ed.) *Explorations on Martha Rogers' Science of Unitary Beings*, Norwalk, CO: Appleton-Century-Crofts, 1986.

45. Newman, M. *Health as Expanding Consciousness*, New York: National League for Nursing Press, 1994.
46. Parse, R.R. Quality of life: sciencing and living the art of human becoming, *Nursing and Science Quarterly*, 1994, **7**, 1, 16–21.
47. Wheatley, M. *Leadership and the New Science: Learning about Organization from an Orderly Universe*, San Francisco: Berrett-Koehler, 1992.
48. Newman, M.A., Sime, A.M. and Corcoran-Perry, S.A. The focus of the discipline of nursing, *Advances in Nursing Science*, 1991, **14**, 1, 1–6, p. 4.
49. McIntyre, M. The focus on the discipline of nursing: a critique and extension, *Advances in Nursing Science*, 1995, **18**, 1, 27–35.
50. Lamb, G.S. and Stempel, J.E. Nursing case management from the client's view: growing as insider-expert, *Nursing Outlook*, 1994, **42**, 1, 7–13.
51. Wheatley, *op. cit.*
52. American Association of Critical-Care Nurses *A Model for Differentiated Nursing Practice*, Washington: AACN Press, 1995.
53. Sharp, L.F. and Priesmeyer, H.R. Tutorial: Chaos theory – a primer for health care, *Quality Management in Health Care*, 1995, **3**, 4, 71–86.
54. Fielding Institute. Research Methodologies, unpublished report, Santa Barbara, CA, 1992.
55. Ford-Gilboe, M., Campbell, J. and Berman, H. Stories and numbers: coexistence without compromise, *Advances in Nursing Science*, 1995, **18**, 1, 14–26.
56. Harding, S. Is there a feminist method? In N. Tuana (ed.) *Feminism and Science*, Bloomington: Indiana University, 1989.
57. Ford-Gilboe *et al.*, *op. cit.*
58. Teilhard du Chardin, P. *The Phenomenon of Man*, New York: Harper & Row, 1959.
59. *Ibid.*, p. 172.

CHAPTER SEVEN

Postmodern research and emancipatory feminism

The Eternal Female groan'd!
it was heard over all the Earth. [1]

INTRODUCTION

The final strand of postmodern research I wish to consider is the notion that social change or social emancipation can come about through the act of doing research, that certain approaches to research are, *by their very nature*, productive of change. There are at least two broad approaches to emancipatory social research, both of which arguably predated the postmodern turn in the social sciences. One of these is the self-styled 'new paradigm' school of research, which attempted to 'discuss and develop ways of going about research which were *alternatives* to orthodox approaches, alternatives which would do justice to the humanness of all those involved in the research endeavour'.[2] Developed in the late 1970s, this new paradigm espoused many of the values that would later emerge in the writing of postmodernist philosophers, including a rejection of the positivist-empiricist epistemology, a privileging of subjectivity, a focus on reflexivity, an emphasis on local and contingent knowledge, and, most significantly, a questioning of the power hierarchy between researcher and researched. In many ways, then, the 'new paradigm' researcher *is* a postmodern researcher.

A second and, from a postmodern perspective, more problematic approach to emancipatory research comes from the broad school of feminist methodologies. Feminist theory has always shared an ambivalent relationship with postmodernism. On the one hand, the anti-foundationalism of postmodern philosophy was predated by feminism and its attack on the grand narrative of 'phallocentric', male-dominated society. Thus 'feminism might welcome certain aspects of a postmodern philosophy, suspicious of universals, problematizing the

Subject, as an attack being made on a different front from that engaged directly by feminism'.[3] For some writers, then, 'feminism and postmodernism are natural allies',[4] while others go even further, claiming that feminist theory is no less than 'a type of postmodern philosophy'.[5] On the other hand, however, the relationship is not without its contradictions, two of which will be considered here.

First, there is the problem of anti-foundationalism itself: if the defining characteristic of postmodernism is an incredulity towards metanarratives, that must surely include the metanarrative of feminism. Thus, Sabina Lovibond pointed out that 'one of the first thoughts likely to occur in the course of any historical reflection on feminism is that it is a typically *modern* movement',[6] and as such, it is inconsistent with the postmodern turn. Nancy Hartsock voiced the suspicions of many modernist feminists when she wrote:

> Why is it that just at the moment when so many of us who have been silenced begin to demand the right to name ourselves, to act as subjects rather than objects of history, that just then the concept of subjecthood becomes problematic? Just when we are forming our own theories about the world, uncertainty emerges about whether the world can be theorized. Just when we are talking about the changes we want, ideas of progress and the possibility of systematically and rationally organizing human society become dubious and suspect?[7]

This is particularly problematic for radical feminists such as Shulamith Firestone, who invoked biological differences between women and men in a positive, empowering way to justify the feminist struggle,[8] since, as Fraser and Nicholson pointed out, 'such appeals to biology to explain social phenomena are essentialist and monocausal'.[9] Furthermore, while rejecting the metanarrative of phallocentric masculinity, a number of feminists have themselves detected hidden 'quasi-metanarratives' of race, class and sexuality in much mainstream feminist writing. As Jane Flax has noted, there are a multiplicity of feminisms, and thus, no single standpoint 'which is more true than previous [male] ones'.[10] Clearly, then, Lyotard's call for an attitude of incredulity towards metanarratives can also be seen as demanding an incredulity towards much of the so-called second wave of 'standpoint' and 'radical' feminist theory, although some writers have warned that 'in legitimate critique of some of the earlier [feminist] assumptions we may stray too far from feminism's original project'.[11] The challenge, then, is to theorize a non-essentialist philosophy of gender relations that is still recognizably feminist.

The second contradiction between feminism and postmodernism lies in the more specific rejection by the latter of the particular meta-narrative of the Enlightenment project and its promise of universal emancipation. For Patricia Waugh, then, 'feminism cannot sustain itself as an emancipatory movement unless it acknowledges its found-ation in the discourses of modernity,[12] and as Lovibond pointed out, 'how can anyone ask me to say goodbye to "emancipatory metanarra-tives" when my own emancipation is still such a patchy, hit-and-miss affair?'[13] Similarly, Sandra Harding has noted that 'perhaps only those who have had access to the benefits of the Enlightenment can "give up" those benefits',[14] a view echoed in Usher and Edwards' observation that:

> feminism is itself located in the legacy of the Enlightenment tradition; the latter's emancipatory impulse nurtures the roots both of eigh-teenth- and nineteenth-century feminism and Marxism. Certainly it was not unattractive for women to believe that, even though they have been defined as incapable of self-emancipation in the past, neverthe-less a commitment to the concepts of reason, objective truth and bene-ficial progress through scientific enquiry would eventually lead to an acceptance of their potential and capacity to be regarded as men's equals.[15]

However, they continued by pointing out that it is the very failure of the Enlightenment tradition to 'deliver' on emancipation that prompted many feminists to look to postmodernism for a solution. But what would an emancipatory postmodern feminism look like, and how would it deal with the seeming rejection by postmodernism of all 'isms', including feminism? As Fraser and Nicholson asked:

> How can we combine a postmodernist incredulity toward metanarra-tives with the social-critical power of feminism? How can we conceive a version of criticism without philosophy which is robust enough to handle the tough job of analysing sexism in all its 'endless variety and monotonous similarity'?[16]

For many feminists, this is an important question. Unlike Lovibond, they do not believe that postmodernism can simply be dismissed; instead, it is an 'unavoidable ensemble of new cultural practices and knowledges',[17] which must be faced head-on. However, as I attempted to show in Part I, an acceptance of postmodernism does not necessarily entail the rejection of political or moral positions. Thus, it might be possible to construct what Squiers has termed 'a post-Enlightenment defence of principled positions, without the essentialist or transcendental illusions of Enlightenment thought'.[18] In a similar vein, Patti Lather called for a 'resistance postmodernism':

> that refuses to abandon the project of emancipation and, indeed, positions feminism as much of the impetus for the articulation of a postmodernism that both problematizes and advances emancipatory work.[19]

Other feminists accept the epistemological relativism implicit in much postmodern philosophy, but argue that this is perfectly compatible with feminism, since knowledge does not necessarily lead to emancipation. Thus:

> Just because false knowledge can be used to justify or support domination, it does not follow that true knowledge will diminish it or that the possessor of 'less false' knowledge will be free from complicity in the domination of others.[20]

Emancipatory feminism, from this perspective, is therefore concerned less with the quest for knowledge than with political change, and 'what we – as feminists – want is not truth but *justice*'.[21] This stance, which (along with postmodernism) rejects the promise of ultimate truth 'but does not deny us a political vocabulary, a vocabulary of values',[22] has been variously termed 'politically informed relativism',[23] 'contingent foundationalism'[24] and 'feminist postmodernism'.[25]

As a strand of postmodern research, this feminist postmodernism has some interesting implications, not least of which is that its primary goal is not the generation of knowledge but the facilitation of change, which it shares with certain approaches to action research. Thus, action research is 'the systematic study of attempts to change and improve... practice by groups of participants by means of their own practical actions',[26] and 'the fundamental aim of action research is to improve practice rather than to produce knowledge'.[27] The questions which still remain to be answered are, however: what counts as improvement; who decides whether a situation really has been made better?; and ultimately, is it really possible to reintroduce value judgements and maintain a philosophy that is still recognizably postmodernist? These are the questions that Kathleen Fahy addresses in her essay later in this chapter.

KATHLEEN FAHY ON EMANCIPATORY FEMINISM

The above dilemma is spelt out in the title of Fahy's paper: 'Postmodern feminist emancipatory research: is it an oxymoron?' In fact, there is a potential double oxymoron in this title, which encourages us to ask two questions: first, is there an implicit contradiction in the notion of a postmodern feminism?; and second, can postmodernism deal with issues of emancipation, or are they necessarily rejected along with the Enlightenment project? Fahy addresses each in turn, starting with the second. Thus, she points out that, whereas postmodernism is usually associated with anti-humanism, 'it is possible to be a postmodern researcher without abandoning humanistic ideals'.[28] It is worth pausing for a moment to consider Fahy's deployment of the terms 'humanism' and 'antihumanism'. Humanism can be defined as the belief or attitude emphasizing common human needs and seeking solely rational ways of solving human problems, and whereas postmodernists might therefore accurately be described as anti-humanists, it is not a term that the majority would use to describe themselves.[29] The problem is that, in popular usage, the term 'humanism' has become conflated with 'humanitarianism', so that to be anti-humanist is often thought of as being against the promotion of human welfare. It is ironic, then, that the philosophical strand of postmodernism, which was initiated largely by Lyotard's despair at the anti-humanitarian outcomes of the Enlightenment project (Auschwitz and so on), should have become associated with that same anti-humanitarianism.

Returning to Fahy's claim that it is possible to construct a humanist postmodernism (or a postmodern humanism), she begins by noting that 'some forms of postmodernism actually serve the purposes of resistance and emancipation'. In particular, the study of postmodern notions of power might lead to 'theories about processes of enlightenment and empowerment for both nurses and clients'. Although Fahy does not give any examples, we might consider Foucault's work in this respect, particularly his notion of discourse and the ways in which power relations are determined and controlled through and between discourses. But the difficulty (and this is where the first potential oxymoron raises its head) is in how postmodernism is defined. For Fahy, the central question becomes, 'Is postmodernism the latest stage of the Enlightenment and a continuation of the humanist project, or a rupture with that era and the beginning of a new age?' If the latter, she argues, 'then humanism is dead, and our emancipatory ideals and values along with it'.

However, her own answer is more optimistic: she puts forward the case that postmodernism rejects the Enlightenment narrative without necessarily rejecting the emancipatory ideal,[30] that, in fact, the humanist ideal is itself (in some ways) anti-emancipatory. Thus, 'the postmodern critique of humanism argues that valuing autonomy and individual rights comes at the price of devaluing the rights of community, other animals and the environment'. In particular, Fahy points out, humanists privilege reason over the emotions, which invalidates many of the ways in which women 'know', so that 'the resulting humanist subject turns out not to be a universal "human"; instead, the image is of one particular, culturally constituted form of human subjectivity: the young, strong, white, elite and male'. Furthermore, this self-actualizing, autonomous man has only been able to pursue the humanist project at the expense of woman.

This critique is, of course, the cornerstone of much feminist theory, and a number of solutions have been postulated. For example, radical feminists such as Shulamith Firestone have argued that the reason for the dominance of male over female culture is not because of the adoption of certain philosophical stances such as humanism or capitalism, but because of biology, in particular the biology of reproduction: women's place in the world 'sprang from a biological reality; men and women were created different and not equal'.[31] Thus, since the cause of inequality is biological, so too is the solution: female biology must be changed, and, indeed, modern technology has made the possibility of such a change (through *in vitro* fertilization, for example) much closer than when Firestone first published her book in 1970.

Other early feminist writers took a less radical and more humanist approach, but, according to Fahy, only managed to substitute the grand narrative of the white middle-class male for that of the white middle-class female, which has simply served to alienate these women from other classes and cultures. Thus, Susan Bordo noted that 'there are no common areas of experience' for all women, and that 'the bonds of womanhood is a feminist fantasy borne out of the ethnocentrism of white, middle class academics'.[32]

For Fahy, then, the humanist ideal has tended to promote certain sectors of society at the expense of others, and is therefore not truly emancipatory. She also invokes Foucault's argument that humanistic values have been employed to normalize behaviour, and have thus become a form of subjugation, 'reducing human freedom and eradicating human differences', and extends his critique to research and to nursing, an issue to which I will return later in the chapter.

Fahy then turns her attention to the other potential oxymoron of the possibility of a postmodern feminism. She notes that whereas the so-called second wave of feminists of the 1970s were striving (as we have seen, unsuccessfully) towards a universal theory, the later 'feminists of difference' rejected the notion of an authentic or natural feminine identity, and, with it, the grand narrative of feminism. Fahy cites the American Judith Butler and the French writer Luce Irigaray, both of whom adopted an anti-essentialist view of woman, as examples of this school of feminism. Butler, for example, argued that the gender category of 'woman' is a construct that might actually serve to undermine the feminist project, and attempted to deconstruct the notion of gender as a substantive category.[33] In a similar vein, Irigaray argued that we should not attempt to define 'woman', since to do so is to perpetuate the phallocentric discourse of polarity and opposition. Josette Féral illustrated this point with the observation that French feminists have made no attempt to copy the American strategy of introducing linguistic changes such as 'Ms' or 'her story', since 'to do so would be, in effect, to play into the game of power by assuming once more that woman has no place, except in the lacunae of a discourse which allows some minor nibblings, as long as the implicit foundations of phallo-theo-logo-centrism are never questioned'.[34] Instead, feminists must put the entire discourse into question, 'to renounce, in effect, the identity principle, the principles of unity and resemblance which allow for the constitution of phallocentric society'.[35]

For Irigaray, then, there can be no unitary definition of woman; as the title of her most famous work *The Sex Which Is Not One* suggested, woman should not be conceived as either the double or the opposite of man, but as heterogenous and multiple. As Fahy points out, however, Irigaray at once denied the possibility of unitary, singular subjectivity while at the same time offering 'an invitation to live a free, artistic and individualistic existence'. This, for Fahy, is a contradictory position to hold, since 'even as they deny authentic subjectivity, postmodern feminists end up producing images of an inner, authentic, heroic feminine identity that refuses and challenges all culturally ascribed feminine roles'.

This is the point at which Fahy attempts to resolve the apparent oxymoron of the postmodern feminist: on the one hand, it is contradictory to be both a feminist and an anti-humanist, yet on the other, the supposedly anti-humanist philosophy of postmodernism would appear to have a great deal to offer to feminism. The solution, it seems, is that postmodernism is not so opposed to the values of humanism as it would first appear. Fahy cites Pauline Johnson's view that the postmodern strategy of ironic playfulness is based on the humanist values of authenticity and autonomy,[36] and she might well have added Alison Assiter's observation that 'it need not follow that an autonomous self must be a whole, unified non-fragmented self. The autonomous self... can have unconscious desires and wishes; it can have desires whose form and whose objects may be transformed'.[37]

Having established her claim for a humanist postmodernism, Fahy then goes on to claim that Lyotard was wrong to have rejected humanism in the first place simply because of the atrocities committed in its name. After all, she continues, contemporary humanists also acknowledge and condemn such atrocities, but still maintain the basic humanist values; it is possible, then, to be both a humanist *and* a postmodernist, and hence both a feminist and a postmodernist. Furthermore, Fahy cites a number of feminists, including Lyn Yates, Patti Lather, Jan Sawicki, Chris Weedon, Jane Flax and Laura Kipnis, as advocates of an emancipatory, politically active postmodernism, and aligns herself with this 'oppositional postmodernism' that draws on ironic or ludic postmodernism 'but then adds a form of material intervention aimed at improving social practice'.

The question that Fahy leaves largely unanswered is how this can be possible within a philosophy that rejects any overarching rationale of what might be meant by improvement. Fortunately, we have already explored two answers to this question in the first part of this book. Thus, Lyotard saw the task of resolving the *differend*, the dispute between competing little narratives, as the main role of the philosopher, and argued that it was possible to make judgements between them from the 'metalanguage' of postmodern philosophy.[38] Similarly, Rorty described the liberal ironist, whose 'final vocabulary', like Lyotard's metalanguage, was spoken in the full awareness of its own contingency, but which nevertheless proclaimed its status as the 'best' description of the world, albeit from a rationally indefensible position.[39]

The feminist Alison Assiter offered another solution to the problem of making judgements in a broadly constructivist world. She postulated 'epistemic communities' that shared similarities with Rorty's 'liberal utopia' in that:

> an epistemic community... will be a group of individuals who share certain fundamental interests, values and beliefs in common, for example, that sexism is wrong, that racism is wrong, and who work on consequences of these presuppositions.[40]

The main difference, however, is that whereas Rorty's liberal ironist recognizes that her final vocabulary cannot be defended on the strength of its epistemological superiority, the individuals who make up Assiter's epistemic communities 'are particularly interested in the truth of their views, and in providing evidence for their truth'.[41] Following the work of Sandra Harding, Assiter argued that disagreements between epistemological communities can be settled by a recourse to the criterion of emancipation, that the most emancipatory philosophy is the one we should subscribe to.[42] She claimed that emancipation is the most appropriate criterion for making judgements not only from an ethical perspective, but also epistemologically, and cited Harding's argument for 'strong objectivity' in research,[43] in which the 'true' perspective is the one that is most inclusive of the views of all interested parties, that is, the most emancipatory.

And this is also Fahy's answer: improved social practice is emancipatory social practice. However, when engaging in such practice, whether it be emancipatory nursing or emancipatory research, the practitioner must be aware of the constraints imposed by the discourse of humanism, in particular by the tendency for normalization that places the nurse or researcher in the role of an expert. Thus, Fahy offers a number of guidelines for the researcher. Researchers must be aware of the power differential inherent in the researcher–participant relationship, and develop ways of balancing this. The traditional feminist solution has been to develop reciprocity, which involves a negotiation of all aspects of the relationship, such that boundaries are not determined in advance but are articulated and (re)negotiated at every stage of the process. Furthermore, the researcher should not hide behind her role, but should 'be herself' in a true human-to-human encounter with the research participant, which blurs not only their respective roles, but also the boundaries between formal and personal relationships. Only by this cohesion of rationality and emotion can truly emancipatory research take place.

Postmodern feminist emancipatory research: is it an oxymoron?[44]

Kathleen Fahy

INTRODUCTION

As a nursing researcher who uses feminist emancipatory methods, I have had a methodological struggle with the notion of embracing post-structural theories as part of my practice. This is because both nursing and feminism are based on humanistic ethics while postmodernism is usually equated with anti-humanism.[45] Some have argued that collaboration with postmodern ideas will undermine both scientific and emancipatory aspirations. I disagree with this assertion and claim instead that it is possible to be a postmodern researcher without abandoning humanistic ideals. The critique of humanism has been particularly problematic for emancipatory researchers because the very notion of emancipation is infused with humanistic values. In this paper I plan to redeem the claim that rather than being undermined by postmodernism, some forms of postmodernism actually serve the purposes of resistance and emancipation.

Postmodern notions of power and subjectivity are particularly useful in emancipatory studies to uncover the strategies and tactics of power, submission and resistance. Within nursing, combining postmodern theories and emancipatory practices will help us to see more clearly the organizational structures and the social processes which reproduce medical dominance and nursing submission. These critiques of current health care practices will be grounded in, and validated by, the experiences of researchers and participants. The linking of postmodern theories about power and subjectivity to emancipatory research practices means that we will be able to develop theories about processes of enlightenment and empowerment for both nurses and clients.[46]

The term 'postmodernism' is understood in different ways across the different fields of inquiry. The physical sciences are dominated by chaos theory and quantum mechanics, which see the universe as being constituted by forces of disorder, unpredictability, non-linearity, diversity and instability.[47] For some, postmodernism is primarily about technologies of information: computer simulated environments, cybernetics and hyperspace.[48] Postmodern work in literary theory, history and philosophy is usually referred to as post-structuralism.[49]

Post-structuralism had its beginnings in European, particularly French, philosophy. Until the late 1960s French philosophy was divided between the individualistic theories of phenomenology and existentialism on one end of a continuum, and collectivism theories dominated by Marxism on the other. In opposition to both of these, cultural structuralism arose in the mid-1960s, inspired by the linguistics of Levi-Strauss and Barthes and by Freudian psychoanalysis. Structuralism challenged both phenomenology and orthodox Marxism by 'dethroning the sign from the centre of meaning and displacing consciousness from the centre of subjectivity'.[50] Structuralists advocated a formal system of analysis with rules and conventions which provide a way of examining interactions between the system and its individual elements; in the case of sociology, the social practices by which society and culture relate to and govern the individual. Post-structuralism goes even further by putting language at the centre of social reality. Rather than reflecting reality, post-structuralists argue, language creates it. Post-structuralism links language, subjectivity, social organization and power.[51] Post-structuralists, including Foucault, Lyotard, Baudrillard, Deleuze, Guattari, and Derrida, undermine all previous assumptions and make all knowledges, including structuralism, problematic.[52] According to Smart, post-structuralists:

> call attention and contribute to the crisis of representation... They reveal the fragile and problematic representational character of language, the disarticulation of words and things and the ways in which meaning is increasingly sustained through mechanisms of self-referentiality and thereby deny us access to an independent reality.[53]

The terms 'post-structuralism' and 'postmodernism' are often used interchangeably, but they are not identical concepts; postmodernism is a broader, more inclusive concept than post-structuralism. Some argue that the term postmodernism should have its meaning confined to the larger cultural and aesthetic changes associated with post-industrialism and post-colonialism.[54] However, the conflation of post-structuralism with postmodernism is now accepted as a *fait accompli* and the words can legitimately be used synonymously.[55]

Much of the debate between modern humanists and postmodern thinkers hinges on the particular understanding that each author has of humanism. For emancipatory researchers, the central question becomes: 'Is postmodernism the latest stage of the Enlightenment and a continuation of the humanistic project, or a rupture with that era and the beginning of a new age?'. If we see that postmodernism represents a complete rupture with the Enlightenment, then humanism is dead, and our emancipatory ideals and values along with it. In the next section, I will argue that although humanism has a dark underside which has allowed people to do terrible things while claiming to be humanistic, I do not think that we have to abandon humanism altogether.

POSTMODERN CRITIQUE OF HUMANISM

Humanism is based on values which stress autonomy, integrity, human rights and self-conscious rationality.[56] The postmodern critique of humanism argues that valuing autonomy and individual rights comes at the price of devaluing the rights of community, other animals and the environment. Humanists have been assailed because they have privileged reason over emotions, and this has meant that decisions about the world and how we should live have been made and enacted without reference to emotions, values or relational attachments.[57] In addition, by eliminating feelings and emotions as ways of knowing, many of the ways in which women 'know' have been invalidated. The resulting humanist subject turns out not to be a universal 'human'; rather the image is of one particular, culturally constituted form of human subjectivity: the young, strong, white, elite and male.

The humanist subject, the relatively autonomous man (sic) creating his own destiny, struggling with his fate, making himself, has been purchased at the price of increasing the oppression of women.[58] Only by women assuming all responsibility for child-care, elder care and home care have men been able to be free of their relational responsibilities and therefore able to follow their self-actualizing path. This idealized subject functions as a standard against which diverse lives can be assessed to see if they 'measure up'. This has had negative consequences for women and non-elite men because he or she, who is not like this idealized subject, is judged inferior to and in need of 'guidance', 'normalization' and 'protection' from dominant white males.

The early feminist writers such as De Beauvoir, Mitchell, Millett and Greer, participated in humanism, but instead of the privileged white male as their subject, they substituted the privileged white female. Many women have felt disenfranchised by these feminist theorists' commitments to a particular image of the subject. Like the male humanistic subject, the feminist subject, the liberated woman, acted as a criterion against which other women judged themselves or were judged by others. Lower-class women complained that only privileged women could expect to be able to afford the financial costs of liberation, such as paying others to perform caring functions. In addition, only middle- and upper-class working women, who work within a career ladder, have been in a position to benefit from equal pay. Many women have complained that their lives were distorted or ignored by these early feminist writers. For example, women who wanted to care for their families felt disparaged and alienated. Lesbian women felt excluded by the heterosexist assumptions that underpinned the idealized liberated woman living in equality with a male partner and co-parent. Women of colour, who often feel even more oppressed because of their race than they are because of their sex, have complained of being subsumed by early white feminist theorists who are blind to the oppressiveness of both racism and colonialism.[59]

Humanism is vulnerable to criticism because atrocities have been committed and oppressive social practices have been perfected in its name. The humanist subject, driven by his reason and cut off from his emotions, has been perceived to be 'making a better world', a more civilized, 'advanced', 'happier' one. This image of the subject has functioned as legitimation for the destruction of the natural and social world and the pollution of the environment. In both capitalist and communist countries, humanistic ideals have been used as justification for invading and colonizing other countries and cultures. Humanism was supposed to lead to human emancipation of people, but it has also functioned as a way of normalizing, controlling and oppressing people. Marxism and capitalism have used the humanist subject as a way of prescribing a particular view of what it means to be human. This has been most obvious during the cultural revolution in China when 'normalizing' techniques were used in attempts to impose a particular form of subjectivity on all Chinese people.

Foucault argued that humanistic values have become the ideological vessels through which the norms and expectations of a specific way of life are imposed on individuals, thus reducing human freedom and eradicating human differences.[60] These social ideals take on the force of normative expectations that serve as a set of instructions by which the 'self-made individual' makes him or herself over. Foucault identified a variety of practices, or self-disciplines, that people carry out on their own bodies, souls, thoughts and actions.[61] For example, he claimed that the disciplinary technologies of fitness regimens, diets and self-reflective practices subjugate people by diverting their energies from following their own desires. Instead, they use their energies to normalize themselves, guided by socially approved forms of subjectivity. This normalization usually takes place under the guidance of an external authority figure, for example a psychiatrist, social worker or other expert.

This critique of humanism potentially undermines the emancipatory project of feminist research by placing the researcher in the position of 'expert', and the researched is at risk of being 'normalized' by the research process. This same concern applies to nursing practice, where the nurse may impose his/her 'expert' 'rational' opinions and values on the patient/client, who is expected to conform to these prescriptions about how to be healthy. Nurses who use the system of Nursing Diagnosis and engage in diagnosing and managing client 'problems' are at great risk of this kind of normalizing imposition which, rather than promoting client empowerment, may actually undermine it.

Postmodernism has declared the subject dead. In postmodern parlance, there is no innate, uniquely human subjectivity or set of traits, or best ways of living. The subject of most emancipatory discourses, in contradistinction, is seen as rational, conscious and authentic; herein lies the challenge for emancipatory researchers. Lacan has been an influential postmodern psychoanalytic theorist who argues that there is no true or inner self; that the individual takes on different identities depending upon the people with whom she/he is interacting.[62] Instead of a single, unified and autonomous subject, there are only multiple, socially prescribed subject positions that dictate what we think, feel and say. Like Lacan, Foucault denies that there is an authentic, inherent subject who, humanists believe, struggles against his/her socially ascribed roles.[63] He sees the subject as entirely socially constructed; who we are, he would argue, is the result of the power relations which have shaped who we may and may not be. For Foucault:

> the individual is not conceived as a sort of elementary nucleus, a primitive atom, a multiple and inert material on which power comes to fasten... In fact, it is already one of the prime effects of power that certain bodies, certain gestures, certain discourse, certain desires come to be identified and constituted as individuals.[64]

In his writings on sexuality, Foucault developed the theme of an 'aesthetics of existence'. By this he meant that although society attempts to govern and limit who we may be, individuals have the capacity to act intentionally, and playfully make creative use of any spaces created by and within the governing norms of society. Although this sounds something like the autonomy of humanism, he is not using the idea in the way that humanists mean self-legislating freedom of action; his is a much more modest claim to freedom.

FEMINIST CRITIQUE OF HUMANISM

A number of influential feminist theorists have developed distinctly anti-humanist positions. The feminists of difference, particularly those known as the French Feminists, have been influenced by French male writers and have taken up Foucault's idea of the 'aesthetics of existence'. This is seen, for example in Luce Irigaray's *The Sex Which Is Not One*[65] and Judith Butler's *Gender Trouble*.[66] These feminists use the idea of an 'aesthetics of existence' to reject the notion of an authentic or natural feminine identity that is inherent to all women. Rather, these feminists seek to encourage a subversive attitude to imposed feminine roles. Postmodern feminists have also participated in the critique of humanistic ethics of justice, freedom and autonomy by arguing that there can be no intersubjectively agreed criteria for judging the worth of different ways of living, and this creates some problems for emancipatory researchers. Most challengingly, how could we know what we are striving for in our role as a facilitator of emancipation? Irigaray, like Lyotard,[67] offers no normative criteria for judging what is a good life, the kind of life worth striving for. An ethic of sexual difference, she argues, does not seek any general agreement; instead, it is an invitation to live a free, artistic and individualistic existence.

I argue that it is difficult, if not impossible, to be both a feminist and an anti-humanist. Feminists value human freedom, autonomy and self-conscious reflexivity; these are humanistic values which imply an inner, authentic subject.[68] Patti Lather agrees; she writes that all feminisms appeal to the 'powers of individual agency and subjectivity as necessary components of socially transformative struggle'[69] to bring about women's liberation from unnecessary oppression. The postmodern view of subjectivity has the effect of representing woman as some kind of cultural robot with little self-understanding or freedom of action. Such a view denies women's awareness of what constitutes their own best interests and their agency in making their own choices. As Johnson pointed out, the postmodern strategy of ironic playfulness and 'creative self-realization' is itself based on a version of humanistic values of authenticity and autonomy.[70] Even as they deny any authentic subjectivity, postmodern feminists end up producing images of an inner, authentic, heroic feminine identity that refuses and challenges all culturally ascribed feminine roles.[71] These post-structural theorists, then, are not really that far from the values of contemporary humanists.

Present-day feminists have rejected the notion of a set of universal essential human needs which define what it is to be human. I acknowledge that the individual's identity is, to a large extent, discursively and historically constituted, resulting in an identity that is both fragmented and dynamic. I reject, however, the postmodern notion that there is no true or authentic self. With many other feminists, I maintain a belief in the 'inner' self who is protected from the distortions of taking on the masks of multiple, culturally available subject positions. The self I am describing is *a priori*, natural and innate. This belief in the inner, or true, self is consistent with Jung's notion of the Self[72] and with many religious conceptions of the soul and the spirit. Following Jung's understanding, the Self is buried in the unconscious and is full of creative potential. The process of socialization, of fitting people for multiple roles in society, involves repressing and thwarting the Self. These roles, or subject positions, are based on expectations, rewards and punishments.[73] Being fully absorbed in enacting our given subject positions alienates us from who we really are and who we might become. It is this 'authentic self' who is vital to the emancipatory project. The goal of emancipatory feminism is to facilitate the emergence of the true self and the creative project of human becoming. Rosemary Parse[74] and Jean Watson[75] promote a similar goal for nursing practice, believing that only through clients becoming more fully who they are can they find healthful ways of living.

Johnson claimed that the postmodern critiques of humanism have been based on a caricature of an outdated form of humanism. Contemporary humanists, she argued, also acknowledge the damage that has been done in the name of humanistic values but, Johnson says (and I agree), this is not a reason to abandon those values.[76] Contemporary humanists, for example, Jurgen Habermas,[77] Angus Heller and Ferenec Feher,[78] see humanism and the Enlightenment project as unfinished and unfinishable. The humanistic values underpinning the Enlightenment represent virtues that enliven our struggles to free ourselves from our own ignorance and prejudices. Present-day humanists acknowledge the need to value human plurality and difference. It is not contradictory to claim that all humans should be accorded freedom and justice, and simultaneously support the value of individual personalities and lifestyle differences. It is not contradictory to claim, on the one hand, to value the human capacity for reason while, on the other, valuing emotion and intuition which arise from our feelings. Feelings are bodily experiences, whereas emotions and intuitions involve both bodily sensations and cognitive processes that make meaning of these sensations.[79] When we can link our feelings, emotions, intuitions and reason together, then we are in the best position for deciding what to do and how to proceed in life. Embracing both humanistic and the postmodern ideas creates a productive synergy from which to theorize.

EMANCIPATORY POSTMODERNISM?

I do not agree with those who have argued that postmodernism is incompatible with politically motivated inquiry. In this negative view, postmodernism is a form of disinterested, intellectual amusement. For example, Gitlin claimed that postmodernism 'neither embraces nor criticizes, but beholds the world blankly, with a knowingness that dissolves feeling and commitment to irony'.[80] In other words, it is not the business of postmodern inquiry to be politically committed or active, merely to observe and comment. In another, but related critique, postmodernism, by promoting introverted, intrinsically gratifying contemplation, may obstruct activism by inducing lethargy. This is why postmodernism has been called the 'opiate of the intelligentsia'.[81] Habermas warns that postmodernism fosters nihilism, relativism and political irresponsibility.[82] He encourages us to remain true to the intentions of the Enlightenment, particularly to the belief in human reason to solve human problems.

Postmodernism has created a crisis for all the human sciences, including the feminisms. The concept of crisis, however, represents both danger and opportunity. The foregoing discussion, by focusing on the postmodern, highlighted the dangers for emancipatory researchers. There are many feminist scholars, however, who support the notion that, rather than undermine emancipatory feminism, postmodernism helps to sharpen the critical edge of research. Lyn Yates, for example, claimed that 'at its best postmodernism is challenging, politically aware, disruptive, creative, rightly suspicious of authority and grand claims'.[83] Patti Lather aligned herself with those 'attempting to create a cultural and adversarial postmodernism, a postmodernism of resistance'.[84] Jana Sawicki, a philosopher who calls herself a Foucauldian feminist, asserted that it 'is compatible with feminism as a pluralistic and emancipatory radical politics'.[85] Chris Weedon affirmed that postmodernism offers feminists opportunities to avoid dogmatism and the reductionism of single-cause analysis, to produce knowledge from which to act.[86]

Jane Flax recommended that those seeking to use postmodernism in the name of emancipatory politics should use the growing uncertainty with Western thought to think more about how we think,[87] and Laura Kipnis, claimed that feminism is 'the paradigmatic political discourse of postmodernism'.[88]

I have been arguing that it is possible to conduct emancipatory research within postmodernism because the postmodern critique of Enlightenment assumptions is not a total refutation of all our humanistic values upon which we base our hope for changing the present towards a better future. Kincheloe and McLaren are among those who argue that humanism and our emancipatory aspirations have not been undermined by postmodernism.[89] Instead, they claim, some postmodern theories actually strengthen emancipatory research and theory. They distinguish two theoretical strands within postmodernism. One they term 'ludic postmodernism' (meaning playful or derisive), and the other 'oppositional postmodernism'. The work of postmodern 'ludic' theorists like Lyotard, Derrida and Irigaray, are characterized by playfulness and focus on differences. While they function to criticize culture, they do not propose ways of changing culture for the better. It is ludic postmodernism that is the target for most of the criticisms given above.

The second strand of theoretical postmodernism identified by Kincheloe and McLaren, which they termed 'oppositional, or resistance, postmodernism', may draw on the theories of ludic postmodernism, but then adds a form of material intervention aimed at improving social practice. 'In this way, postmodern critique can serve as an interventionist and transformative critique of Western culture'.[90] I align myself with oppositional postmodernism and value the synergy that this creates between critical feminism and postmodern discourses. Critical feminism provides postmodern discourses with a normative foundation, and postmodern discourses unsettle grand theories, promote creativity and undermine the notion that there is one 'true' version of social reality.

IMPLICATIONS FOR NURSING RESEARCH PRACTICE

I return now to a postmodern challenge presented earlier: that humanism presents a version of subjectivity to which individuals are supposed to conform, and that this normalization usually takes place under the guidance of an external authority figure. This critique of humanism potentially undermines the emancipatory project of femi-

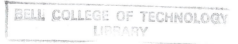

nist nursing research by placing the researcher in the position of 'expert', and the researched is at risk of being 'normalized' by the research process. In response to this real concern, feminist researchers need to be continuously conscious of the power differential that exists between themselves and participants. Finding ways to balance this power differential is one of the key principles underpinning feminist methodological procedures.[91] This principle is given expression in research practice by fostering reciprocity, which means building-in ways to promote mutuality, equality and sharing between the researcher and the participants. Reciprocity involves negotiating all aspects of the relationship. There are no predetermined boundaries between researcher and participant; these have to be articulated and negotiated. The researcher must essentially 'be herself' in the relationship and not hide behind the role of nurse or researcher. Reciprocity involves a true human-to-human encounter with all the emotionality that this implies. Reciprocity means blurring the boundaries between formal and personal relationships so that the lives of the researcher and 'subject' often become entwined, as in friendship.[92]

CONCLUSION

This paper arose in response to a methodological struggle that I experienced as I began to incorporate post-structural theories into my emancipatory research practice. I have argued that postmodernism is compatible with politically motivated, humanistically based inquiry, and simultaneously asserted that the postmodern critique of humanism, which exposes its dangers, requires emancipatory researchers to defend their practices, both in relation to research participants and in the ways in which the subject is theorized.

Postmodern notions of power and subjectivity can strengthen the theoretical power of emancipatory studies. The creative tension generated by post-structural theories and emancipatory ideals help us to conceptualize embodied experiences and to uncover the strategies and tactics of power, submission, resistance and change in more useful ways than modernist theories allow. I have argued that some forms of postmodernism serve the purposes of researchers who want their practices and their theories to contribute to changing the present towards a better future. These emancipatory theories should, I have argued, be based on a colligation of reason and emotion; on an embodied rationality. Ultimately, it is not reason, logic or intellectual analysis that controls human decisions or gives our lives their meaning and direction. One must feel, emotionally and biologically, a sense of active excitement about being alive in order to create and protect a life worth living. Helping research participants and/or nursing clients to achieve this state is far more challenging and far less arrogant than providing prescriptions about what research participants or nursing patients 'should' do in order to be happy and healthy.

NOTES

1. Blake, W. *A Song of Liberty*, 1793.
2. Reason, P. and Rowan, J. *Human Inquiry: A Sourcebook of New Paradigm Research*, Chichester: John Wiley, 1981, p. xi, original emphasis.
3. Docherty, T. *Postmodernism: A Reader*, New York: Harvester Wheatsheaf, 1993, p. 366.
4. Assiter, A. *Enlightened Women: Modernist Feminism in a Postmodern Age*, London: Routledge, 1996, p. 4.
5. Flax, J. Gender as a Social Problem: In and For Feminist Theory, *Journal of the German Association for American Studies*, 1986.
6. Lovibond, S. (1990) Feminism and postmodernism. In T. Docherty (ed.) *Postmodernism: A Reader*, New York: Harvester Wheatsheaf, 1993, p. 394, original emphasis.
7. Hartsock, N. Foucault on power: a theory for women? In L. Nicholson (ed.) *Feminism/Postmodernism*, New York: Routledge, 1990, pp. 163–4.
8. Firestone, S. *The Dialectic of Sex*, New York: Bantam, 1970.
9. Fraser, N. and Nicholson, L. Social criticism without philosophy: an encounter between feminism and postmodernism, *Theory, Culture and Society*, 1988, **5**, 2–3, 373–94.
10. Flax, *op. cit.*, p. 37.
11. Barrett, M. and Phillips, A. *Destabilizing Theory: Contemporary Feminist Debates*, Cambridge: Polity Press, 1992, p. 6.
12. Waugh, P. Postmodern theory: the current debate. In P. Waugh (ed.) *Postmodernism: A Reader*, London: Hodder & Stoughton, 1992, p. 190.
13. Lovibond, *op. cit.*, p. 395.
14. Harding, S. *Feminism and Methodology: Social Science Issues*, Milton Keynes: Open University Press, 1987.
15. Usher and Edwards, *op. cit.*, p. 20.
16. Fraser and Nicholson, *op. cit.*, p. 393.
17. Ebert, T. Review of '*Feminism/Postmodernism*', *Women's Review of Books*, 1991, **8**, 4, 24–5, p. 24.
18. Squiers, J. *Principled Positions: Postmodernism and the Rediscovery of Value*, London: Lawrence & Wisheart, 1993, p. 2.
19. Lather, P. Staying dumb? Feminist research and pedagogy with/in the postmodern. In H.W. Simons and M. Billig (eds) *After Postmodernism: Reconstructing Ideology Critique*, London: Sage, 1994, p. 102.

20. Flax, J. The end of innocence. In J. Butler and J.W. Scott (eds) *Feminists Theorise the Political*, London: Routledge, 1992, p. 458.
21. Gill, R. Relativism, reflexivity and politics: interrogating discourse analysis from a feminist perspective. In S. Wilkinson and C. Kitzinger (eds) *Feminism and Discourse*, London: Sage, 1995, p. 178.
22. *Ibid.*, p. 178.
23. *Ibid.*, p. 178.
24. Butler, J. Contingent foundations: feminism and the question of 'postmodernism'. In J. Butler and J.W. Scott (eds) *Feminists Theorise the Political*, London: Routledge, 1992.
25. Fraser and Nicholson, *op. cit.*
26. Ebbutt, D. Educational action research: some general concerns and specific quibbles. In R.G. Burgess (ed.) *Issues in Educational Research: Qualitative Methods*, Lewes: Falmer Press, 1985, p. 156.
27. Elliott, J. *Action Research for Educational Change*, Milton Keynes, Open University Press, 1991.
28. All unreferenced quotations are from Fahy's section in this chapter.
29. Postmodernists are still concerned with (re)solving human problems, and are critical of the means rather than the ends of humanism. Most would therefore prefer the terms 'anti-essentialist' (a rejection of the notion of 'essences' such as truth, self or identity) or 'anti-subjectivist' (against the idea of the autonomous subject) to describe their stance.
30. In Rorty's words, 'to retain Enlightenment liberalism while dropping Enlightenment rationalism': Rorty, R. *Contingency, Irony and Solidarity*, Cambridge: Cambridge University Press, 1989, p. 57.
31. Firestone, *op. cit.*, p. 16.
32. Bordo, S. Feminism, postmodernism and gender scepticism. In L.J. Nicholson (ed.) *Feminism/Postmodernism*, London: Routledge, 1990, p. 133.
33. Butler, J. *Gender Trouble, Feminism and the Subversion of Identity*, London: Routledge, 1990.
34. Féral, J. The powers of difference. In H. Eisenstein and A. Jardine (eds) *The Future of Difference*, New Brunswick: Rutgers University Press, 1980, p. 91.
35. *Ibid.*, p. 91.
36. This can certainly be seen in the work of Richard Rorty, for whom, it will be recalled, ironism was the strategy that reconciled the seemingly opposed philosophies of postmodernism and liberalism.
37. Assiter, *op. cit.*, p. 109.
38. Lyotard, J.-F. *The Differend: Phrases in Dispute*, G. Van Den Abeele (trans.) Manchester: Manchester University Press, 1988.
39. Rorty, *op. cit.*
40. Assiter, *op. cit.*, p. 82.
41. *Ibid.*, p. 82.
42. Compare this with Rorty's similar defining criterion of a liberal community, which is that cruelty is the worst thing that one person can do to another. Rorty, *op. cit.*

43. Harding, S. *Whose Science? Whose Knowledge? Thinking from Women's Lives,* Oxford: Oxford University Press, 1991.
44. First published in *Nursing Inquiry,* 1997, **4**, 27–33.
45. See, for example, Giddens, A. *Sociology,* Cambridge: Polity Press, 1989. Johnson, P. *Feminism as Radical Humanism,* St Leonards, NSW: Allen & Unwin, 1994.
46. Johnson, *op. cit.*
47. Gleick, J. *Chaos,* London: Cardinal, 1987.
48. For example, Baudrillard, J. The precession of simulacra. In B. Wallis (ed.) *After Modernism: Rethinking Representation,* Boston: David Godive Publishing, 1984, pp. 253–81. Poster, M. Foucault, the present and history, *Cultural Critique,* 1988, **8**, 105–21.
49. Boyne, R. and Rattsini, A. (eds) *Postmodernism and Society,* London: Macmillan, 1990.
50. Grosz, E. *Sexual Subversions: Three French Feminists,* North Sydney: Allen & Unwin, 1989, p. 10.
51. *Ibid.*
52. Richardson, L. Writing: a method of inquiry. In N.K. Denzin and Y.S. Lincoln (eds), *Handbook of Qualitative Research,* Thousand Oaks, CA: Sage, 1994, pp. 516–29.
53. Smart, B. *Postmodernity,* London: Routledge, 1993, pp. 20–1.
54. See, for example, Boyne and Rattsini, *op. cit.*; Lather, P. *Getting Smart: Feminist Research and Pedagogy with/in the Postmodern,* New York: Routledge, 1991.
55. See, for example, Boyne and Rattsini, *op. cit.*; Lather, *op. cit.*; Smart, *op. cit.*
56. Johnson, *op. cit.*
57. *Ibid.*
58. Pateman, C. *The Sexual Contract,* Cambridge: Polity Press, 1988.
59. Hill Collins, P. *Black Feminist Thought: Knowledge, Consciousness, and the Politics of Empowerment,* Boston: Unwin Hyman, 1990.
60. Foucault, M. Introduction. In P. Rabinow (ed.) *The Foucault Reader: An Introduction to Foucault's Thought,* New York: Pantheon Books, 1984, pp. 3–29.
61. *Ibid.*
62. Grosz, E. *Jacques Lacan: A Feminist Introduction,* London: Routledge, 1990.
63. Foucault, M. *The History of Sexuality,* Volume 1, New York: Vintage/Random House, 1984.
64. *Ibid.,* p. 98.
65. Irigaray, L. *The Sex Which Is Not One,* Ithica, NY: Cornell University Press, 1985.
66. Butler, J. *Gender Trouble: Feminism and the Subversion of Identity,* London: Routledge, 1990.
67. Lyotard, J.-F. *The Postmodern Condition,* Manchester: Manchester University Press, 1984.
68. Nash, K. The feminist production of knowledge: is deconstruction a practice for women? *Feminist Review,* 1994, **47**, 65–76.
69. Lather, *op. cit.,* p. 28.

70. Johnson, *op. cit.*
71. Irigaray, *op. cit.*; Butler, *op. cit.*
72. Jung, C.G. *On the Nature of the Psyche*, Princeton, NJ: Princeton University Press, 1960.
73. Butler, J. *Bodies That Matter: The Discursive Limits of 'Sex'*, Routledge: New York, 1993.
74. Parse, R. Human becoming: Parse's theory of nursing, *Nursing Science Quarterly*, 1992, **5**, 1, 35–42.
75. Watson, J. *Nursing: Human Science and Human Care*, Norwalk, CT: Appleton-Century-Crofts, 1985.
76. Johnson, *op. cit.*
77. Habermas, J. *Postmetaphysical Thinking: Philosophical Essays*, Cambridge: MIT Press, 1992.
78. Heller, A. and Feher, F. *The Grandeur and Twilight of Radical Universalism*, New Jersey: Transaction Publishers, 1991.
79. Stanley, L. and Wise, S. *Breaking Out Again: Feminist Ontology and Epistemology*, 2nd edn, London: Routledge, 1993.
80. Gitlin, T. Postmodernism: roots and politics. In I. Angus and S. Ghally (eds), *Cultural Politics in Contemporary America*, Routledge: London, 1989, p. 347.
81. Dowling, W.C. *Jameson, Althusser, Marx: An Introduction to the Political Unconsciousness*, Ithica, NY: Cornell University Press, 1984.
82. Habermas, J. *The Theory of Communicative Action – Lifeworld and System: A Critique of Functionalist Reason*, Volume 2, Cambridge: Polity Press, 1987.
83. Yates, L. Postmodernism, feminism and cultural politics, or if master narratives have been discredited, what does Giroux think he is doing? *Discourse*, 1992, **13**, 1, p. 124 .
84. Lather, *op. cit.*, p. 1.
85 Sawicki, J. Identity politics and sexual freedom. In I. Diamond and L. Quinby (eds) *Feminism and Foucault: Reflections on Resistance*, Boston: Northeastern University Press, 1988, pp. 177–91.
86. Weedon, C. *Feminist Practice and Poststructuralist Theory*, Oxford: Basil Blackwell, 1987.
87. Flax, J. Postmodernism and gender relations in feminist theory, *Signs*, 1978, **8**, 2, 202–23.
88. Kipnis, L. Feminism: the political conscience of postmodernism? In A. Ross (ed.) *Universal Abandon: The Politics of Postmodernism*, Minneapolis: University of Minnesota Press, 1988, pp. 149–66.
89. Kincheloe, J.L. and McLaren, P.L. Rethinking critical theory and qualitative research. In N.K. Denzin and Y.S. Lincoln (eds) *Handbook of Qualitative Research*, Thousand Oaks, CA: Sage, 1994, pp. 138–57.
90. *Ibid.*, p. 144.
91. See, for example, Lather, *op. cit.* Stanley and Wise, *op. cit.* Reinharz, S. *Feminist Methods in Social Research*, New York: Oxford University Press, 1992.
92. Reinharz, *op cit.*

CHAPTER EIGHT

Postmodern research and the ironist nurse researcher

General Knowledge is Remote Knowledge;
it is in Particulars that Wisdom consists and Happiness too.[1]

INTRODUCTION

The methodologies outlined and discussed in the previous four chapters can be seen as spanning a continuum of postmodern positions from Walker's 'counter-hegemonic' stance of oral narrativity, through Rolfe's incorporation of writing into the narrative tradition, and Koerner's assimilation of postmodernism into the discourse of science (or rather, the expansion of science to include postmodernism), to Fahy's reconciliation of humanism with postmodernism (albeit, a reconciliation that maintains the oppositional stance of resistance). In this final chapter, I wish to consider how the postmodern ironist researcher outlined at the end of Part I might function in the real world of nursing and health service research.

It will be recalled from Chapter Three that the postmodern ironist researcher accepts epistemic relativism, the view that knowledge is socially constructed, and is therefore contingent on the individual knower, on the language game that she is currently playing, or on the broader culture in which she operates, while at the same time rejecting judgemental relativism. To take Rorty's example as an illustration of this position, words like 'knowledge' and 'truth' function in much the same way as words such as 'me' and 'here'; we all share an understanding of what is meant by them, although the objects or concepts to which they refer might well be different in each case, depending on who utters them. When two people simultaneously say 'Give it to me', we see no contradiction or other logical problem over the use of the word 'me' as referring to two different people; instead, we recognize that we are being asked to make a choice. Similarly, when two people say, respectively, 'X is true' and 'X is not true', the ironist would not necessarily question the use of the word 'true', nor would she see any logical contradiction between the two statements; as in the previous example, she would see the two statements as an invitation to make a choice. Furthermore, the choice cannot be made from some third 'metaposition' from which she is able to judge the 'real' truth of X, since there is no metaposition, no grand narrative of truth. All that she can say is that, from her perspective, she will choose to regard X as either true or not true according to whatever suits her needs at the time.

What is important, however, and what separates the postmodern ironist from the postmodern relativist, is that the ironist is at least able to choose whether or not to regard X as true, whereas the out-and-out relativist can only say something like 'It depends on which way you look at it.' The ironist's choice, however, is contingent and tentative: she chooses a particular option on the understanding that she cannot logically or empirically defend that option; it merely fits better with the language game that she is currently playing.[2] Furthermore, when she offers her own 'truths' to others, she does so on the understanding that she cannot justify them with reference to a metanarrative; she cannot say 'This is universally true, and you must therefore believe it', since the values and logic of her language game will be different from those of other language games. She cannot, therefore, construct a rational argument for her position; she cannot, to quote Rorty, 'argue for this suggestion on the basis of antecedent criteria common to the old and the new language games. For just insofar as the new language game really is new, there will be no such criteria.'[3] All she can do is:

> to redescribe lots and lots of things in new ways, until [she has] created a pattern of linguistic behaviour which will tempt the rising generation to adopt it, thereby causing them to look for appropriate new form of nonlinguistic behaviour, for example, the adoption of new scientific equipment of new social institutions.[4]

Thus, a poet cannot convince a mathematician by reasoning or argument that poetry deals in higher truths than mathematics, since the language she would need to use would be alien to the mathematician (and vice versa). Not only would the idea of poetry being somehow 'true' be hard for the mathematician to accept (since they both have a different conception of what is meant by truth), but, more fundamentally, the mathematician's notion of what counts as proof would lead her to reject all the arguments put forward by the poet as mere rhetoric. All the poet can do is to offer her poems in the hope that the mathematician is moved by them to the extent that she is tempted to learn the language of poetry.

When this postmodern ironist position is applied to research, it results in a number of interesting implications, three of which will be considered here. First, the aim of ironist research is not to uncover universal truths; rather than discovering a fixed and unchanging monolith of knowledge, the ironist researcher is, to use an analogy, shining a small torch from a particular angle on part of that monolith. Unlike the out-and-out relativist, then, the ironist is not denying the existence of a real(ist) world, nor is she necessarily claiming that we can never 'know' that world, simply that we can never know that we know it. My particular torch might reveal 'the whole truth and nothing but the truth', whereas the view that yours reveals might be so partial and distorted as to be unrecognizable, but there is no objective grand narrative, no accurate plan of the monolith, from which to make such a decision. Furthermore, we cannot even tell from our partial views whether there is one monolith or many, whether it is static or moving, stable or ever changing. Even staunch upholders of the scientific method recognized this difficulty. As Popper said of his method of hypothetico-deductivism, 'we test for truth, by eliminating falsehood. That we cannot give a justification – or sufficient reasons – for our guesses does not mean that we may not have guessed the truth; some of our hypotheses may well be true.'[5] It is just that we can never know for sure. The aim of ironist research, then, is not to disclose some absolute truth, but to throw some light on the situation, to illuminate a dark corner.

Second, once we let go of the idea that research can provide us with a guarantee of truth, we are no longer slaves to the tyranny of method. From the positivist perspective, a rigid adherence to research methods is a guarantee of both internal and external validity. So, for example, internal validity, 'the degree to which an instrument measures what it is supposed to be measuring',[6] is closely related to the construction and administration of that instrument. As soon as the researcher modifies the instrument or administers it in a non-standard way, the validity of the entire research project is compromised. Even in qualitative research, where terms such as 'credibility' and 'trustworthiness' are preferred to 'validity', it is still expected that standardized methods will be employed, such that 'using an inappropriate method to answer a research question may result in loss of generalizability, increased cost, and invalidity'.[7] Furthermore 'method slurring' is generally frowned upon, and 'such mixing, while certainly "do-able", violates the assumption of data collection techniques and methods of analysis of all the methods used. The product is not good science; the product is a sloppy mishmash'.[8] Similarly, for the positivist, external validity or generalizability can only be assured by following rigid sampling criteria, so that the sample is statistically representative of a wider population.

For the scientific researcher, then, the aim of research is to produce knowledge, and this aim can only be assured by a close adherence to the rules of method; what, how and to whom she addresses her research question are all rigidly prescribed. For the ironist, however, the aim is not to generate knowledge but to illuminate, and she recognizes that all attempts at illumination are partial, and that none can offer a 'better' illumination than any other. Thus, validity is not an issue, and all methods have something to contribute, including many that might not be considered by scientific researchers, such as those discussed in the previous chapters; each illuminates a different aspect of the 'truth', and the more perspectives we have, the more rounded and complete is our picture.

Third, and most importantly, the aims and methods of postmodern ironist research lead inexorably to a subjectivist position in which we are forced to make choices without the benefit of a metanarrative to provide us with a rationale for those choices. The postmodernist would, of course, claim that *all* researchers, including modernists and positivists, are in a similar position, but that they do not realize it; they believe that the scientific method underwrites their chosen methodology and makes it superior to the postmodern methodologies of (say) reflective writing or feminist emancipatory research. From the postmodern perspective, however, it is this blind assumption of superiority that renders traditional scientific research not merely one little narrative among many, but an *inferior* little narrative. The postmodernists argue that science takes itself too seriously; in believing that it holds all the answers, it relinquishes its claim on any answers that it might have had. In contrast, the playful or ironic stance of the postmodernist, who recognizes that her answers are, at best, partial and tentative, provides a more rounded picture of the real world. As Philips, writing 'pre-postmodernism' in the early 1970s, put it:

> Play, by freeing us from a heavy dependence on method, may enable us to confront the world without the scientific 'blinders' required for membership in the sociological [and scientific] community. Play may not only give free rein to the imagination, intuition and creative urges, but may help us see more clearly.[9]

For the postmodern ironist, then, research is a game, one of many language games, in which the rules and terminology only apply within that particular game. The findings of the research are therefore tentative and contingent, and only apply within that particular game. What research tells us depends on which game we choose to play, and we choose in the knowledge that we might not have made the best possible choice; nevertheless, we *must* choose.

CLAIRE PARSONS ON THE IRONIST NURSE RESEARCHER

Qualitative or interpretivist methodologies are usually seen as offering greater flexibility and scope for such choice at every stage of the research process, and it is therefore not surprising that most of the contributors to this book have promoted postmodern research as an alternative to the modernist paradigm of quantitative research, and have enlisted the qualitative paradigm as being more or less sympathetic to their cause. In a similar vein, Parsons, in the discussion that follows, distinguishes between what she refers to as nomothetic science (that is, research that enables generalization from a sample of cases to a global theory) and the 'ideographic understanding'[10] of qualitative research (that is, the concern for unique aspects of individuals). For Parsons, then, social research is concerned with expressing either the collective voice of the large group or the multiple voices of its individual constituents. However, while the qualitative approach 'is not founded on a singular paradigm or theoretical position', and is therefore most readily identifiable with the postmodern turn, she also recognizes that the postmodern critique is probably more damaging to qualitative research methodologies than it is to the modernist quantitative paradigm.

The problem, as Parsons sees it, lies with the dual crises of legitimation and representation. For modernist science, these issues are not problematic: legitimation is dealt with through a number of rigorously controlled validity and reliability checks, whereas representation simply requires conformity to a rigid model of the scientific write-up. Furthermore, there is a certain internal consistency about these various checks and rules, such that they can only be attacked by refuting the entire paradigm of scientific method. While postmodern writers are quick to attack the scientific paradigm as a metanarrative (that is, as *the* method of research), the status of quantitative research as a little narrative (that is, as one method among many) is largely unassailable, since, by the postmodernists' own criterion, the language game of quantitative research cannot be critiqued by other incommensurable language games. Thus, the quantitative paradigm is, on its own terms, relatively successful in its attempt to 'construct abstract statements about social actors through large groups, randomly selected and never met, observed, spoken to, interacted with or interpreted in the light of the context from which they speak'; from the postmodern perspective, we cannot critique the means of quantitative research, but only its ends.

In contrast, qualitative researchers play language games very similar to those of postmodernists, believing that 'it is better to concentrate on the detail, complexity and contextually grounded meanings that can account for the experience and activities of a small number of individuals' (that is, with individual little narratives), and while its ends are commendable, its means are far more vulnerable to the postmodern critique. The difficulty is that the qualitative researcher is usually concerned with capturing some aspect of the 'lived experience' of the participant, yet Parsons acknowledges the postmodernist claim that such experience 'is already mediated through the political ideology of a particular sociocultural language game and is refracted yet again through the lens of the researcher in the final account'. Thus, she continues, 'the idea that a [qualitative] researcher can somehow elicit and/or observe experience directly, then analyse that and reformulate it into a sophisticated analysis that presents an authentic, clear statement of the everyday world of research participants, finds its epitaph in postmodernism'. This failure to achieve its ends has been referred to as the 'crisis of legitimation', and poses enormous problems; as Parsons notes, 'the absence of a true (valid) base upon which to construct social theory threatened the core of qualitative research'.[11]

A second and related crisis for qualitative research has been termed the 'crisis of representation'; this is concerned with issues of how the multiple voices of the research participants are to be represented and heard in the final text. This crisis is compounded by the additional problem, highlighted above, of the impact and influence of the researcher herself on the situation she is researching. Thus, 'the collecting of fieldwork data is not a matter of collecting or gathering data (as if units called "data" are lying around to be garnered), but is instead a selective process guided by the research question and the political ideology of the mind of the researcher and the researched'. If, as we saw in earlier chapters, even the 'hard' scientific researcher influences the situation she is observing, then the qualitative social researcher, who is dealing with living, thinking human beings, clearly cannot help but have a profound impact on the data she collects. Writing up, then, is a subjective, interpretive process of presenting the equally subjective and interpretive process of collecting data; as

Parsons puts it, it is 'the final report, article, story, or "tales of the field" that may render an impressionistic, confessional, realist, critical, literary, analytic, grounded theory, or other form of artful and political interpretive account'.

The most usual response of researchers to this crisis of representation is to write reflexively, that is, to attempt to write themselves (and their respondents) into the research report; in the words of Michael Billig, to 'repopulate the text',[12] so that (in Parsons' words) the researcher 'becomes a conduit for multiple voices to be expressed, while adding her or his voice to the data, results and conclusions'. However, there are two difficulties that reflexive writing largely fails to address: first, as Parsons points out, 'there remains the necessity to speak to policy makers in the bureaucratic language that they understand'; and second, there is the problem of the rejection by postmodernists of the notion of the autonomous 'subject' and the subsequent denial of the possibility of empowerment. The latter issue has been discussed extensively in earlier chapters, so I shall focus here on the problem of reconciling the modernist, nomothetic approach to research (particularly to the research report) demanded by policymakers and administrators, with a reflexive postmodern approach that allows the voices of individuals to be heard.

To some extent, Parsons sees this problem as a temporary (albeit fairly long-term) one for nursing; it will partly be resolved as more and more graduate nurses who are familiar with the new reflexive approaches to research come into the workforce. This is a promising (albeit, perhaps, optimistic) conclusion, particularly in the light of the current call from the popular press for a return to 'work at the bedpan level'[13] and a rejection of 'the nihilistic, politically correct gibberish that has disfigured social sciences'.[14] In contrast to the growing demand for a 'dumbing-down' of nursing, then, Parsons envisages an eventual 'smartening up' of nurses and a consequent acceptance of Phillips' 'nihilistic, politically correct gibberish' of (presumably) postmodernism. Furthermore, nurses have an affinity for small-scale, applied studies in the practice setting, are well placed to hear and represent the voices of their patients, and 'are therefore receptive to the postmodern concerns about those who study the experience, meaning and context of everyday lives'. However, there remains a tension, at least in the medium term, between these postmodern, reflexive sensibilities and 'the continuing demand to report objectively on a reality other than the researcher's'.

Parsons' recognizes what Lyotard referred to as the *differend* in action, the unfair judgement between the two (in Lyotard's terminology) 'phrase regimens' of modernist and postmodernist research according to the rules and values of the former.[15] Her solution to this dilemma is a perfect example of the 'playful' ironist researcher at work/play. Thus, she strives to 'straddle modern and postmodern imperatives by accommodating selected postmodern insights to inform and interact with what are essentially modern research designs'; that is, to employ a postmodern sensibility while conducting and writing up (largely) modernist research. And as we have seen, the realization of the flaws and limitations of modernist research, that it is, in effect, not a metanarrative but merely one little narrative among many, gives her an advantage over her more positivist colleagues. Whereas, from a postmodern perspective, *all* researchers are working within one or other little narratives, Parsons' little narrative is what Rorty referred to as 'ironic' (see Chapter Three), that is, a narrative that is aware of its own contingency. This ironic awareness puts Parsons at an advantage by allowing her to function within an imperfect system in which an adhesion to the rules does not guarantee the legitimation of the findings. She is thus able to bend the rules, adopting modernist methods where it suits her cause, 'while increasing [her] own consciousness of the paucity of such methods, and of the ideological and non-definitive nature of all research'.

So, for example, Parsons continues the practice of 'writing the voices of participants into the research report', but not for the usual modernist reasons of ensuring validity, such that 'the voice of the researcher's analysis articulates with the voices of the research parti cipants', since such a practice is intrinsically flawed. Instead, she allows the voices to 'speak of their own interests, meanings and values, as opposed to those of the researcher'. It is not an ideal situation, but as she (ironically) points out, 'it is all we have at present'. Furthermore, it subverts the seemingly objective scientific research report in favour of the subjective goal of the empowerment of the participants, so that the researcher becomes 'a small part of a larger movement that will forge the new revisionist techniques for research in time for a new century in which emancipatory approaches to research will undoubtedly have a stronger hold'. Like Fahy, then, Parsons sees the ultimate goal of postmodern research as emancipation, and leaves us with a tantalizing vision in which 'the distanced, objective, scientific researcher is beginning to fade in the shadow of the critical and more action-oriented (and even activist) researcher'.

The impact of postmodernism on research methodology: implications for nursing[16]

Claire Parsons

FROM MODERN TO POSTMODERN

In the era of what has retrospectively become known as 'modern' science, researchers established relatively stable criteria for assessing the rigour (reliability, validity, generalizability) and therein the quality or 'scientific merit' of research. While science had earlier established its 'gold standard' for quality control through the experimental method, researchers who applied quantitative methods to social research co-opted the gold standard as being equally applicable to the social arena. Here, the preference is for nomothetic science based on large, randomly selected samples of populations from which 'findings' are extrapolated that are said to represent and predict the behaviours of all those in the population that match on a limited number of characteristics, for example, the same range of socio-demographic and illness characteristics.

Qualitative methodologists were usually those disenchanted with the assumptions and abstract techniques used to generate statistics that were thought to speak for all 'similar' groups, and instead turned to methods that they believed enhanced the quality of their research. They sought the 'deep' understanding, or 'thick description,[17] an emic (internal) and ideographic understanding of a range of complex characteristics and contextualized actions (behaviours and meanings) of a group of people or 'cases'. Methods included small-scale studies in which 'in-depth' interviewing would often be used to gain the thick description, followed by the taking of research (synthetic interpretations of their 'realities') back to the participants for verification. The process was intended to provide a validity check for the research account (as is the practice in most ethnographic, phenomenological and other qualitative approaches). Furthermore, ensuring that social theorizing was grounded in the empirical data of everyday life was itself a control to prevent speculative theory, and this contributed to the validity (and even reliability) of qualitative theorizing. Despite

179

these and other mechanisms to provide some equivalence in rigour to that established in science, many qualitative researchers continued to be concerned about the extent to which researchers could truly understand their participants (through their 'data collection' procedures) or represent the world of 'the other' (through interpretive analysis), and to what extent there could (or should) be any boundary between the researcher and the research participants if understanding, interpretation and even a degree of emancipation, were to be realized.

Today, qualitative methodologies offer a range of data gathering and interpretive techniques while giving no primacy to any particular approach. Unlike quantitative research, qualitative research is not founded on a singular paradigm or theoretical position, and while this releases research discourse from the straightjacket of positivism that is seen to silence competing voices, qualitative researchers have continued to struggle with the fostering of multiple voices from research outset to outcome. The creative search for criteria that constitute rigorous research in qualitative design has generated different criteria for different methodologies. Thus, qualitative researchers have not established a gold standard applicable to assessments of rigour across all qualitative research.

POSTMODERNISM AND THE CRISES OF LEGITIMATION AND REPRESENTATION

Postmodernism, defined by Denzin and Lincoln as a philosophical posture 'that privileges no single authority, method or paradigm'[18] in understanding and interpreting the social world, has since had a major impact on academic research, as it has reformulated the two lingering doubts in scholarship. These are sometimes referred to as: (i) the crisis of legitimation (how can we be certain of the accuracy and authenticity [truth] of the representations we gather in the data collection [construction] process when traditional notions of validity or reliability are being questioned in contemporary research?); and (ii) the crisis of representation (how should researchers write about those they study?).

The crisis of legitimation

The attraction of qualitative research for many is that those who apply its techniques, do so in the belief that it is better to concentrate on the detail, complexity and contextually grounded meanings that can account for the experience and activities of a small number of individuals, than to construct abstract statements about social actors through large groups, randomly selected and never met, observed, spoken to, interacted with, or interpreted in the light of the context from which they speak.

As part of the effort to get closer to understanding the individuals studied, the researcher taking a qualitative approach has often tried to capture directly aspects of human 'experience'. However, the 'experience' of the participants is already mediated through the political ideology of a particular sociocultural language game and is refracted yet again through the lens of the researcher in the final account. Experience is therefore not studied directly, or elicited, but is already created in the various layers of oral and written text. This is not a new insight – the early phenomenologists recognized this dilemma – but it has increasingly constrained the expectations of postmodern researchers when reading authoritative claims. The idea that a researcher can somehow elicit and/or observe experience directly, then analyse that and reformulate it into a sophisticated analysis that presents an authentic, clear statement of the everyday world of research participants, finds its epitaph in postmodernism.

Furthermore, the researcher's account (the research report) is constrained by the intention and value of research. That is, the research process and outcome are tempered by whether the research is intended to facilitate the sharing of experiences (telling a story), influence policy (evaluate life contexts and reconstruct them for the bureaucratic mind in order to mobilize social resources), or be emancipatory (assist participants to deconstruct their 'experience and expressivity' in order to construct them anew and act to enhance their own life situation). Each engages different methods or techniques and intentionally generates different research outcomes. Thus, critical feminists may seek emancipatory ends through assisting women to deconstruct texts as speech or the written word so they can see the patriarchal constructs of everyday speaking, while cultural studies theorists may use methods strategically to reveal how race, class and gender have been constructed so that these groups can learn to resist local structures of domination.[19]

While qualitative researchers surrendered reliability (repeatability), they championed validity, and bathed in the glow of detailed and accurate accounts of their research participants' lives. However, when attention focused on human experience as not being an essence, or commodity, amenable to being captured firsthand, but was itself mediated by an ideologically imbued language, then the absence of a true (valid) base upon which to construct social theory threatened the core of qualitative research.

The perplexity evoked by abandoning traditional criteria for evaluating accuracy and the broad application of findings (validity, reliability, generalizability), while failing to provide indisputable alternatives, constitutes the crisis of legitimation. While poststructuralists continued to focus on the deconstructing of authoritative accounts of history as archaeologies (a retrospective critique of written texts of academics and non-academics alike), postmodern thinkers, who also had an affinity for deconstruction, contributed to both retrospective and contemporary ways of conducting research while offering tentative strategies for accommodating the arguments regarding 'truth' and 'writing about reality'. Hence, postmodern researchers have developed alternative criteria for evaluating their work, such as 'credibility, adequacy, confirmability, verisimilitude, emotionality, personal responsibility, an ethic of caring, transferability, dependability, political praxis, multivoiced texts, and dialogues with subjects'.[20] Those who have co-opted the mantle and standards of modern science regard the alternative criteria as a dilution, or abandonment, of rigour and reason, surrendering to merely speculative and relativist propositions about the nature of human existence, experience and behaviour.

Of course, the crisis of legitimation merges with the crisis of representation as the processes of developing research questions, sampling, data gathering and analysis all influence what emerges as the final research account or report.

The crisis of representation

During the 1970s, while the UK and USA sociologists were pioneering the exploration of the boundaries of reflexive writing[21] (bridging the reflexivity of consciousness and the reflexivity of representation), it was to be anthropologists such as Marcus and Fischer,[22] Turner and Bruner,[23] Clifford and Marcus,[24] Geertz[25] and Clifford[26] who were to break the mould in writing style. The concept of reflexivity, a term that first explained the relationship between consciousness and reflexive moments in thought mediated by language and then the relationship between the biographical time and place (including geographic place, ethnicity, culture, gender, class) of the researcher and researched, was regarded as integral to the research processes and was co-opted and amplified in the rhetoric of postmodern speaking. The notions of reflexivity and the more traditional term, intersubjectivity, assisted theorists to address the problem of the researcher reading herself or himself into researcher narratives, or reports, about their own research findings.

These anthropologists were also to bring generic insights into the meaning and value of such social science and humanities icons as class, gender and culture. Critical feminism and culture theory were two postmodern styles that took up the gauntlet and provided new vistas bringing renewed attention to objectivity, reliability and validity in research. In this light, interpretation seemed to have more substance than grounded and empirical 'raw' data, as researchers met the crises head on and demonstrated how often and to what extent research participants deceive researchers and downright lie (Stoller and Olkes[27] give an example of this) and therefore the researcher cannot rely on the research interview or observation alone to generate an understanding of social life.

It was clearly recognized that fieldwork required different skills and insights from that of writing or representing the real world of social actors. The postmodern writer revealed the distance between fieldwork and the writing up of that data that requires a comprehension of the interpretive moments that bridge field records, description and explanatory statements about the people studied. For postmodernists, this process must be recognized and digested as distanced from any pretensions about producing objective findings, recognizing instead that research is a profoundly subjective process. Indeed, closer scrutiny of fieldwork revealed that the collecting of fieldwork data is not a matter of collecting or gathering data (as if units called 'data' are lying around to be garnered) but is instead a selective process guided by the research question and the political ideology of the mind of the researcher and the researched, a process that merges both fieldwork and writing. Distinctions blur under the weight of the researcher's own historical, biographical, class, cultural, ethnic, genderized, and ideological preconceptions, and therein the politics and ethics of the research pact.

Arising out of this conundrum are numerous articulate debates that have challenged different dimensions of representation, among which those from non-Western cultures that have recently gained some ascendancy (see readings in culture theory and critical feminism) where researchers have convincingly argued against the colonizing of their world-views, the misrepresentation of the world of women and the world of other cultures by white, middle-class male and female academic researchers. Women of colour, disabled and lesbian women destabilized white, middle-class feminist notions of women's place and time. Cultural studies, an interdisciplinary approach that merges critical theory, feminism and poststructuralism[28] identified the mediating processes of politics, ideologically impregnated mass communication, and state approved science, as means for the control of knowledge and constructions of reality for the oppressed.

What we see emerging here are multiple theoretical stances and methods for approaching research that compete for the high ground of claims to research rigour. Emerging from each of these is the final report, article, story, or 'tales of the field' that may render an impressionistic, confessional, realist, critical, literary, analytic, grounded theory, or other form of artful and political interpretive account.[29] Some current qualitative researchers believe in an almost solipsistic premise, that there is no singular interpretive truth, but skirt solipsism by developing shared rules for evaluating particular interpretations. Even the pragmatic and applied arena of 'health programme evaluation', that today relies heavily on qualitative techniques, has developed its own criteria for evaluating its field of interpretation. These include allowing the multiple voices of constituents, health workers, administrators and policy makers to be heard. Thus, a health programme evaluator becomes a conduit for multiple voices to be expressed, while adding her or his voice to the data, results and conclusions to inform health policy. Nevertheless, there remains the necessity to speak to policy makers in the bureaucratic language that they understand. Most still ask the positivist and political means-ends questions: 'what do we know about "this" group of people, their needs and behaviours?'; 'given particular circumstances, what can we predict they will do?'; and 'what cost-effective strategies can we implement to get them to meet our objectives?' (for example health screening to reduce future demand on the health dollar).

LIMITATIONS OF THE APPLICATION OF POSTMODERN THEORIZING TO RESEARCH

Postmodernism, with its call to facilitate and allow individuals to tell their own stories, to identify their own issues and find their own solutions beyond the activities of the researcher, is predicated on an old notion of 'rational man', and an active and articulate self. What remains problematic here is that many of the oppressed do not create a sense of order in their lives, a coherent life story, or self-image. Many have no coherent conception of their own existence, at least not as it is understood in Western culture. These are typically Western, middle-class, assumptions that have been challenged in the writings of women of colour[30] and disabled women in a male-defined culture.[31] The philosopher Sandra Harding, who has reviewed transitions in social science epistemologies and methodologies,[32] challenged the postmodernist agenda for applied research, while Komarovsky[33] and Hawkesworth[34] challenged the postmodern critical stance toward subjectivity and intersubjectivity between researcher and researched, and the social construction of people's lives through a research posture that can paralyse the research endeavour. That is, they questioned whether in postmodern research it is at all possible to report research that has any veracity or adequacy. As Hawkesworth argued, to be left in the realm of relativism is to be left disempowered and with the *status quo*. After all, empowerment requires the reconstruction of people's lives in frameworks that indicate ways to develop and implement strategies for change. Empowerment denies relativism and demands the privileging of one viewpoint over another.

The postmodern invective against what is called 'colonized speaking' and the demand for constellations of perspectives and language styles in representation that offer a spectrum of discursive voices focused on any particular research question or issue, offers important insights but is difficult to integrate into current research when issues and policy, say, in the health arena, move quickly in contrast to the glacial speed of understanding the impact of postmodernism on the historical generation of 'knowledge'. Those in the health industry, whether policy maker, bureaucrat, administrator, educator or practitioner, seek change, purportedly to enhance the quality of lives of others, on a different time and space trajectory than those who author the more academic debates. Thus, real people's lives move at a faster pace than authorships that often attend to a bygone era, or to a future with multidimensional challenges that have yet to be documented as research process.

Thus, the postmodern era is bedevilled with insight, innovative and tentative methods and techniques, a reappraisal of epistemologies and ontologies, and contradiction. Meanwhile, researchers must get on with the activities of research that, for many, straddle modern and postmodern praxis.

IMPLICATIONS FOR NURSING RESEARCH

While most nurse researchers are employed by universities, they usually remain close enough to the practice setting to discover and build theory out of the voices of real people in the everyday world. For all that these university-based nurse researchers are often criticized by their practitioner colleagues for writing abstract articles seemingly unrelated to practice, some are pioneering new ways of thinking about health, illness and nursing practice (see Afaf Meleis's work on culture or Judith Parker's on the postmodern body). While Street is not a nurse, she has made a marked contribution to the field of critical ethnography as applied in nursing.[35]

The criticism about academic nurses writing incomprehensible theoretical articles predates the abstruse lingua franca of poststructuralist and postmodern theorizing. In the past, theory has mostly been developed from practical, everyday data; however, the language used is usually alien to nurses in the clinical setting. This divide will be bridged as more university graduate nurses comprise the nursing complement of hospital and public health settings. The new generation of nursing research and academic writing that reflects the postmodern influence will represent the world differently, more precisely and hopefully in less turgid language.

As nurse practitioners become nurse researchers, they will increasingly ask other questions about research, such as: 'Is there any such thing as "authoritative speaking" that presents a more legitimate or "expert" version of reality than any other?'; or 'Is the researcher's account a more accurate or insightful account of a particular aspect of everyday life than the research participants' own accounts?' Here, nurses are asking the same questions other novice researchers ask, but the sensibilities the practice nurse brings to research might advantage the acquisition of the critical reflexivity required by the postmodern genre.

To explain, nurses are not usually armchair theorists, but like to conduct their research in the practice setting, whether that setting be hospital or community, and are therefore closer to the realities of practical living and dying, everyday mundane experiences, however defined. Nurse researchers increasingly have a propensity for qualitative research and are already positioned to hear and represent the voices of the other, that is, they usually study patients as members of the community (whether local, national or international) or other health colleagues. Many nurses have an affinity for small scale, applied studies that attempt to understand the detail of the experience of individuals. They are therefore receptive to the postmodern concerns about those who study experience, meaning and contexts of everyday lives. Unlike most social scientists, it is they who deal most intensively with the used and abused. It is they who interact with individuals when they are being their least theatrical selves (as illness often strips away the layers of social guises) and listen to the modest stories (confessions, divulgences) of the oppressed and oppressor alike. Through clinical practice, nurses are steeped in the mundane and complex world of 'ordinary folk' living 'ordinary lives', although not necessarily 'normal' lives, as they participate in dimensions of the wash of humanity: from archbishops and ministers of the crown to the housewife, farmer, sex worker, homosexual, addict and the mentally disturbed. It is an experiencing of the mundane that the sociologist, anthropologist, political scientist, philosopher, economist or other social researcher is simply not privy to.

Of course, nurse researchers will conduct their research according to the requirements of their research endeavours, producing exploratory writings, using exploratory methodologies for applied research, or traditional modern research approaches. However, if the researcher is answerable to a funding agency, then a report on findings is required and articles usually need to be published presenting methods and findings. It is not the norm to produce a report that is multivoiced, open-ended and remains relativistic; rather, some conclusions need to be drawn so as to present the requisite authoritative statement about 'what was found'. The tension remains between liberating techniques of postmodernism and the continuing demand to report objectively on a reality other than the researcher's. What, then, is a useful strategy that nurse researchers might adopt, at least to enhance their reflexivity in research?

As a researcher answerable to several funding bodies, I straddle modern and postmodern imperatives by accommodating selected postmodern insights to inform and interact with what are essentially modern research designs (to which most researchers answerable to funding agencies are shackled). I reach for insights into the reflexive dimensions of consciousness, researcher-researched intersubjectivity, and reflexivity in writing, to the extent that I am not merely a voyeur of the world of those I seek to understand and empower through the force of a deconstructing argument. Of course, the term 'empower' has a different level of meaning here than that used in the overtly emancipatory research approaches. However, I cannot escape the authoritative statements in which current research is ensnared, or entirely avoid the generalizations in creating patterns in human existence as I see it (interpret it). I am often in the position of being able to influence policy, and take the opportunity to speak through research (and other means) in what is essentially positivist language and through modernist methods write at one level while increasing my own consciousness of the paucity of such methods, and of the ideological and non-definitive nature of all research. As I move from research report to research report there is little time to write the more reflexive articles in the post-modern tenor, but as I move into a new research programme I find I am not untouched by the influences of postmodernist critiques. I seek ways to integrate modernist methods with these critiques. In doing so, I am a small part of a larger movement that will forge the new revisionist techniques for research in time for a new century where emancipatory approaches to research will undoubtedly have a stronger hold. As Denzin and Lincoln write, 'a politics of liberation must always begin with the perspectives, desires, and dreams of those individuals and groups who have been oppressed by the larger ideological, economic, and political forces of a society, or a historical moment'.[36] This is the commitment to empowering others (and in so doing, empowering self) that I and many others researching the health field make. It is a commitment that nurses, already familiar with a tradition of subordination to Medicine in particular and patriarchy in general, often find they make willingly.

Another way in which I straddle modern and postmodern research strategies is continuing the qualitative research practice of writing the voices of participants into the research report. In the past, this has been done so that the reader can see for herself or himself whether the ensuing analysis is a true and plausible (valid) representation of the world of the other. It has always been a selective and therefore partial representation to illustrate, or illuminate, aspects of an argument. This is one of the more traditional steps of legitimation (validation) as the voice of the researcher's analysis articulates with the voices of the research participants. Nurse researchers can continue to use this strategy while exploring the specific postmodern critiques of the extent to which these voices speak of their own interests, meanings and values, as opposed to those of the researcher. However, there are also ethical issues associated with this imperative to represent the voices of the participants. Take, for example, the issue of research confidentiality. In my current research in the field of women's health and among people living with HIV/AIDS, it is important to delete all identifiers, such as names and addresses of participants, from tape recordings and transcripts (both of which are to be stored for 5 years). However, that does not go far enough. It also includes deleting the names of partners, children, neighbours, doctors they visit, and even the veterinarian that the family dog is taken to and the dog's name. Even so, my experience has shown that people can still identify the participant and therefore the narrative must be distorted further, enough to make the narrative useful to illustrate a point of argument yet be fully protective of the participant. This distortion to make the story completely abstract is usually crucial in arenas such as HIV/AIDS. Yet the postmodernist would argue against such researcher interference, against the distortion of the participant's voice. This is the sort of dilemma the postmodernists have yet to confront.

While postmodernists work on new techniques to establish veracity, plausibility and credibility in applied qualitative research accounts while including the requirements of ethical research, nurses too may contribute to such developments. In this way, nurse researchers will continue to link their theorizing (despite critiques about colonized, sociopolitical speaking by researchers) to concrete, empirical, or grounded data (however flawed) upon which they can substantiate conclusions they draw from their research. It is all we have at present. For in the final analysis, research, as it is conducted in the 1990s, remains largely modernist and requires an authoritative account to report research findings, however tentatively stated. In summary, currently, the only avenue for moderating authoritative claims regarding such findings is to continue to allow the multiple voices, the multiple perspectives, to be revealed through the final report (albeit often cleaned of all identifiers and clues to a particular participant's reality) and, where possible, to disclose the researcher's interests and standpoints (class, culture, gender and so on).

There are benefits for both nurse practitioner and nurse researcher in exploring existing postmodern debates to sharpen their own critical consciousness. The nurse researcher will increasingly identify dimensions of the reflexive nature of researcher and participant intersubjectivity and the reflexive moments of research interaction. Because of their vantage point in interacting intensively at multiple levels and in an enduring way with people from all walks of life, nurses are well positioned to take up many of the challenges of postmodern critique and integrate them into the orthodoxy of current research methods and in their application in the field.

The crisis of representation for any researcher resides in the attention they give to critical reflection that is learned (or not) over many years of research experience. The distanced, objective, scientific researcher is beginning to fade in the shadow of the critical and the more action-oriented (and even activist) researcher. This is despite the hallmark of current qualitative research being uncertainty, exploratory, and a cacophony of inherent contradictions. A new era is emerging in which nurses will see irrevocable changes to the research enterprise and to the application of research in practice settings.

NOTES

1. Blake, W. *The Last Judgement*, 1818.
2. Rorty, as a self-confessed pragmatist, would go further by claiming that she chooses the option that is of more practical use to her: Rorty, R. *Contingency, Irony and Solidarity*, Cambridge: Cambridge University Press, 1989.
3. *Ibid.*, p. 9.
4. *Ibid.*, p. 9.
5. Popper, K.R. *Objective Knowledge*, rev. edn, Oxford: Clarendon Press, 1979, p. 30.
6. Polit, D.F. and Hungler, B.P. *Nursing Research: Principles and Methods*, 5th edn, Philadelphia: J.B. Lippincott, 1995, p. 353.
7. Field, P.A. and Morse, J.M. *Nursing Research: The Application of Qualitative Approaches*, London: Chapman & Hall, 1985, p. 15.
8. Morse, J.M., *Qualitative Nursing Research: A Contemporary Dialogue*, rev. edn, Newbury Park: Sage, 1991, p. 15.
9. Phillips, D.L. *Abandoning Method*, London: Jossey-Bass, 1973, p. 163.
10. All unreferenced quotations are from Parsons' section in this chapter.
11. It is interesting to note that Lyotard recognized a similar crisis in modernist *quantitative* research, but does not address the (arguably) more pressing issue for qualitative research raised by Parsons: Lyotard, J.-F. *The Postmodern Condition*, Manchester: Manchester University Press, 1984.
12. Billig, M. Sod Baudrillard! Or ideology critique in Disney world. In H.W. Simons and M. Billig (eds) *After Postmodernism: Reconstructing Ideology Critique*, London: Sage, 1994, pp. 150–71.
13. Brian Sewell, writing in the *London Evening Standard*. Cited in Payne, D. The knives are out for P2000, *Nursing Times*, 1999, **95**, 4, 14–15.
14. Melanie Phillips, writing in the *Daily Mail*. Cited *ibid.*
15. Lyotard, J.-F. *The Differend: Phrases in Dispute*, Manchester: Manchester University Press, 1998.
16. First published in *Nursing Inquiry*, 1995, **2**, 22–8.
17. Geertz, C. *The Interpretation of Culture*, New York: Basic Books, 1973.
18. Denzin, N. and Lincoln, Y. *Handbook of Qualitative Research*, Newbury Park: Sage, 1994, p. 15.
19. *Ibid.*, p. 14.
20. *Ibid.*
21. Sandywell, B., Silverman, D., Roche, M., Filmer, P. and Phillipson, M. *Problems of Reflexivity and Dialectics in Sociological Inquiry: Language Theorising*

Difference, London: Routledge & Kegan Paul, 1975. Blum, A. *Theorising*, London: Heinemann Educational Books, 1974.

22. Marcus, G. and Fischer, M. *Anthropology as Cultural Critique: An Experimental Moment in the Human Sciences*, Chicago: University of Chicago Press, 1986.

23. Turner, V. and Bruner, E.M. *The Anthropology of Experience*, Urbana, IL: University of Illinois Press, 1986.

24. Clifford, J. and Marcus, G.E. *Writing Culture: The Poetics and Politics of Ethnography*, Berkeley: University of California Press, 1986.

25. Geertz, C. *Works and Lives: The Anthropologist as Author*, Stanford, CT: Stanford University Press, 1988.

26. Clifford, J. *The Predicament of Culture: Twentieth Century Ethnography, Literature and Art*, Cambridge, MA: Harvard University Press, 1988.

27. Stoller, P. and Olkes, C. *In Sorcery's Shadow: A Memoir of Apprenticeship among the Songhay of Niger*, Chicago: University of Chicago Press, 1987.

28. Denzin and Lincoln, *op. cit.*, p. 15.

29. Van Maanen, J. *Tales of the Field: On Writing Ethnography*, Chicago: University of Chicago Press, 1988.

30. Spivak, G. *In Other Worlds: Essays in Cultural Politics*, London: Routledge, 1988. Mohanty, C. Under Western eyes: feminist scholarship and colonial discourses, *Feminist Review*, 1988, **30**, 60–8. Green, R. The Pocohontas perplex: the image of Indian women in American culture. In E. Dubois and V.L. Ruiz (eds) *Unequal Sisters: A Multi-cultural Reader in US Women's History*, Calgary: Detselig, 1990, pp. 15–210. Garcia, A.M. The development of Chicana feminist discourse 1970–1980, *Gender and Society*, 1989, **3**, 217–38.

31. Fine, M. Passions, politics and power: feminist research possibilities. In M. Fine (ed.) *Disruptive Voices*, Ann Arbor, MI: University of Michigan Press, 1992, pp. 1–25.

32. Harding, S. Conclusion: epistemological questions. In S. Harding (ed.) *Feminism and Methodology: Social Science Issues*, Bloomington: Indiana University Press, 1987, pp. 181–90.

33. Komarovsky, M. The new feminist scholarship: some precursors and polemics, *Journal of Marriage and the Family*, 1988, **50**, pp. 585–93.

34. Hawkesworth, M. Knowers, knowing, known: feminist theory and claims of truth. In M.R. Malson, J.F. O'Barr, W. Westphal and M. Wyer (eds) *Feminist Theory in Practice and Process*, Chicago: University of Chicago Press, 1989, pp. 327–51.

35. Street, A. *Inside Nursing: A Critical Ethnography of Clinical Nursing Practice*, Albany: State University of New York Press, 1992.

36. Denzin and Lincoln, *op. cit.*, p. 575.

Project 2001: nursing in the third millennium

Improvement makes strait roads,
but the crooked roads without Improvement are roads of Genius. [1]

WHY NOT POSTMODERNISM?

It is tempting at this point in the book to offer not only a summary, but also a synthesis, some kind of model or theory of postmodern nursing. However, if you have read this far, you will realize the futility of such an attempt. First, of course, postmodernism resists such theory-building; it mistrusts grand narratives that attempt to tell 'big stories', including the grand narrative of postmodernism itself. Second, there is in any case no discernible big story, no single account that would do justice to the many strands of postmodern nursing that have been presented and discussed in this book, let alone the almost infinite number that space (and ignorance) have required me to omit. Even within the broad scope of postmodernism, the individual narratives or phrases (to use Lyotard's terminology) arise from different regimens (or what Wittgenstein referred to as different language games), so disputes between them cannot be settled rationally. Third, if there is no grand narrative, there is no 'end'; that is, there is no single aim to which all nurses are aspiring, and hence no end-point when that aim is achieved. A neat and simple closure to this book is clearly not possible.

Having spent most of the book attempting to answer the question 'why postmodernism?', I will end by considering the question 'Why not postmodernism?' If postmodernism is, as I have claimed, such a good thing for nursing, why does it continue to be looked upon with such mistrust? The problem, I will attempt to show, lies not with the practice of nursing, but with the theoretical discourse; my argument is that the language of nursing is constructed in such a way as to make postmodernist nursing practice, research and education not so much un*do*able as un*think*able. Furthermore, this state of affairs has not arisen by

192

accident; instead, the modernist discourse has shaped the language of nursing in such a way that any challenges to it are made to appear absurd or irrational. Those with the power to define what counts as good practice, research and education have used that power to ensure that only modernist practice, research and education are seen as valid. As we shall see, one of the key tasks of the postmodern discourse of nursing is concerned with exposing the ways in which modernism has left its opponents without a voice by labelling them as unacademic; but, of course, postmodern nursing finds itself labelled as one of those 'unacademic' (and hence voiceless) opponents. This leaves postmodernist nursing with the seemingly impossible task of lifting itself by its own bootstraps.

PROJECT 2000: MODERNIST NURSING AND ACADEMIC DISCOURSE

It was not until the late 1980s that the discourse of nursing made its bid for academic respectability in the UK with the introduction of Project 2000. Project 2000 was a new curriculum initiative that took first-level nurse training into higher education, while at the same time strengthening its theoretical base; in the terminology of the educationalist Hazel Bines, it was a move from pre-technocratic to technocratic education.[2] According to Bines, the ethos of technocratic education is based on three principles: first, the development and transmission of a systematic knowledge base comprised mainly from established academic disciplines such as the social and natural sciences; second, the interpretation and application of that knowledge base to practice, usually involving theoretical models; and third, supervised practice in carefully selected placements to ensure that the theory is being properly applied.

Clearly, however, Project 2000 was intended to be far more than simply another curriculum initiative. The expectation was that it would have a profound influence on the entire discipline of nursing, and that a technocratic curriculum would eventually result in a technocratic profession in which practice was based as far as possible on the application of scientific knowledge, theory and research. Project 2000, then, was the first step towards a complete and coherent approach to nursing theory, practice, education and research, a new academic paradigm for nursing in which theory takes supremacy over practice. I will henceforth use the term 'Project 2000' to refer not just to the educational curriculum, but also to the entire modernist, technocratic paradigm.

This modernist turn to academic theory is evident in all aspects of Project 2000 nursing. In research, it can be seen in the privileging of large-scale quantitative studies from which generalizable theories can be generated, over smaller qualitative projects and individual case studies. In education, it can be seen in curricula structured so that students are first taught theory and then encouraged to apply it to practice in carefully organized and supervised practicums, rather than in the traditional apprenticeship model or the more recent reflective models, in which practical experience comes first and leads to the generation of theory. In the clinical setting, it can be seen in the drive towards evidence-based practice rather than practice based on experience and expertise.

Ironically, Donald Schön criticized what he called this 'technical rationality' paradigm as being unsuitable for practice-based disciplines well before Project 2000 was introduced,[3] pointing out that 'what aspiring practitioners most need to learn, professional schools seem least able to teach'.[4] Schön graphically encapsulated this problem as follows:

> In the varied topography of professional practice, there is a high, hard ground overlooking a swamp. On the high ground, manageable problems lend themselves to solution through the application of research-based theory and technique. In the swampy lowland, messy, confusing problems defy technical solution. The irony of this situation is that the problems of the high ground tend to be relatively unimportant to individuals or society at large, however great their technical interest may be, while in the swamp lie the problems of greatest human concern. The practitioner must choose. Shall he remain on the high ground where he can solve relatively unimportant problems according to prevailing standards of rigor, or shall he descend to the swamp of important problems and nonrigorous inquiry?[5]

Arguably, pre-technocratic nursing took place in the swampy lowland, but had no tools or conceptual frameworks with which to address the 'messy confusing problems' that it encountered there, while technocratic Project 2000 nursing is trying to haul itself out of the swamp by denying the importance (or even the existence) of such problems. Furthermore, by attempting to establish itself as a grand narrative (that is, as *the* way rather than as *a* way), technocratic nursing is denying practitioners the choice that Schön outlined above. Nurses 'descend to the swamp of important problems and nonrigorous inquiry' at their peril, since practice based on such non-rigorous inquiry is by definition not evidence based, and therefore not to be condoned. From the high, hard ground of the grand narrative of technocratic nursing, all clinical problems must be addressed by the application of rigorously generated evidence (preferably from randomized controlled trials), and any problem that cannot be resolved in this way is quietly swept under the carpet. This applies not only to the 'little problems' of messy day-to-day practice, but also to the 'big problems' such as the gap between theory and practice. Since this is not a problem that can be successfully addressed by the application of technocratic methods (which are, arguably, making it worse), the technocrats have attempted to deny that the problem even exists. Indeed, some academics have endeavoured to redefine it so that it is no longer seen as a problem, but an asset;[6] thus, 'a "gap" between theory and practice is not only inevitable and healthy but necessary for change to occur in nursing education'.[7]

PROJECT 2001: POSTMODERNIST NURSING

Postmodernism as a metalanguage

I have claimed, then, that nursing is dominated by a technical rationality paradigm in which statistical research is the gold standard, in which practice is determined by the findings of such research rather than by clinical experience and expertise, and in which the educational curriculum advocates and reinforces the primacy of theory over practice. I also wish to suggest that there is a growing disillusionment with this paradigm, particularly from nurses working in the swampy lowlands of messy, real-life practice, and that this disillusionment is usually articulated in a call for more reflective, holistic, introspective and humanistic approaches to nursing. In some ways, the turn to postmodernism as a rejection of the values and methods of technical rationality is simply the latest phase in the search for alternatives to the dominant paradigm of Project 2000 nursing. I will refer to this postmodernist turn as Project 2001, my vision for nursing in the new millennium.[8]

However, because it is underpinned by a postmodernist philosophy, Project 2001 is fundamentally different from other alternatives such as reflective practice, since it does not seek to replace the technical rationality paradigm with some other paradigm, but to cast an incredulous eye over *all* paradigms. As Lyotard pointed out, all modernist paradigms (what he called narratives or discourses), including that of technical rationality or Project 2000 nursing, are based on phrase regimens or language games that determine what can be expressed within that paradigm, and in what ways.[9] Furthermore, since each paradigm employs its own particular language games, communication between paradigms is difficult, and at times impossible. Disputes between paradigms are therefore usually resolved by the application of power rather than by rational argument, although the power-play is often hidden behind a seemingly rational rhetoric.[10]

Postmodernist Project 2001 nursing is, in contrast, not just another paradigm based on just another phrase regimen or language game; instead, it is an attempt to stand outside *all* paradigms, and is based on a metalanguage, a language that explains how all other language games operate. For Lyotard, the role of the postmodernist lies in uncovering the hidden power-play behind the seemingly rational academic debate, in 'detecting differends and in finding the (impossible) idiom for phrasing them'.[11] Thus, the aim of Project 2001 is not to offer a coherent and self-contained paradigm for nursing that will replace the dominant paradigm of Project 2000, but to 'deconstruct' its modernist philosophy, to show that Project 2000 is not based on a self-evident and infallible truth about the superiority of empirical research, any more than reflective practice is based on a self-evident and infallible truth about the superiority of introspection. Instead, the aim is to show how Project 2000 nursing has manipulated language in such a way that any alternatives to it are made to appear unacademic, or even illogical. The message of Project 2001 is not 'Do it like this', but 'There is no good reason for doing it like that'; it is a message of emancipation from ideology rather than just another ideological message. From this postmodernist perspective, then, the disputes between different nursing paradigms are as much disputes about language and definitions as they are about practice.

Deconstructing research and evidence-based practice

Let us consider, for example, the current issue of research- or evidence-based practice from the perspective of postmodernist Project 2001 nursing. Clearly, the postmodern nurse would not support what she would see as the narrow technical rationality, evidence-based approach of her modernist colleagues. Neither, however, would she wish to fall into the trap of rejecting evidence-based nursing in favour of some non-evidence-based alternative. Instead, she would attempt to demonstrate how the modernists have colonized terms such as 'research' and 'evidence based' to take on a narrow and partial meaning. In fact, many postmodernist nurses would wish to claim that their own practice is research based or evidence based; it is just that they use the words in a rather different sense. For example, Diane Marks-Maran has argued for a postmodernist perspective on evidence-based nursing that attempts to 'step out of the prevailing paradigm of what counts as evidence and seek different answers to human dilemmas or questions that modernism can no longer solve'.[12]

As I have already suggested, the issue is one of power, of the imposition of political authoritarianism (being in authority) over epistemological authoritativeness (being an authority). Thus, just as the academic trend in nursing research was, in the early 1990s, beginning to swing towards an interpretivist qualitative paradigm, the British government used its power to reimpose a traditional positivist definition of research through the Department of Heath (DoH) commissioned *Report of the Taskforce on the Strategy for Research in Nursing, Midwifery and Health Visiting*. The taskforce, chaired not by a nurse but by a Professor of Social Policy, attempted to repress the qualitative paradigm by defining research as 'rigorous and systematic enquiry... designed to lead to *generalizable* contributions to knowledge',[13] that is, as being restricted to studies whose findings can be statistically generalized to a wider population, such as large-scale surveys and controlled clinical trials. Furthermore, anything that does not fall into this category was redefined as 'developmental activities' or 'audit',[14] that is, as not *bona fide* research.

The full impact of this narrow definition becomes clearer elsewhere in the report, where it is pointed out that the government is (and has been for the past three decades) 'the principal source of financial support for research and development in nursing',[15] and any research initiatives not funded by the DoH therefore tend to be 'small-scale project-type work... [which are] not externally funded and are carried out within the individuals' own time'.[16] Also, as the DoH report continues, 'valuable as these are, they tend not to yield generalizable and cumulative knowledge', and, by their own definition, therefore do not qualify as *bona fide* research projects.

This, of course, is a prime example of the relationship between power and knowledge. The DoH has the authoritarian power to define what counts as research: in this case, only externally funded, large-scale projects that are statistically generalizable to a wider population. In addition, since the DoH is one of the very few bodies in a position to fund such substantial projects on a regular and ongoing basis, it is also in a position to decide what research questions will be addressed, how they will be addressed, and who will address them; that is, it has a huge

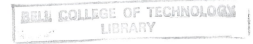

amount of control over the definition and generation of nursing knowledge. Furthermore, since the DoH has also stated that all practice should be based on the findings generated by its own definition of research, it also exerts power and control over nursing practice. Of course, postmodernists and other dissenting academics are free to investigate whatever issues they choose in whatever ways they choose, but, without substantial funding, whatever findings are produced simply will not count as real research, and, in the words of the DoH report, 'must not be seen as a substitute for the generalizable and cumulative research which we would place at the heart of a strategy for advancing research in nursing'.[17] It will not attract funding because it is not real research, and it is not real research because it is not funded.

A similar strategy can be seen in the promotion by the government of the term 'evidence-based practice'. The technical rationality call for research-based nursing has been heard regularly for the past thirty years, but once again there has been a growing concern since the early 1990s in academics and practitioners alike about the benefits of practice based solely on the findings of research.[18] In response, there has been a shift in the rhetoric from *research*-based practice to *evidence*-based practice, although the actual practice to which this new term refers has remained more or less unchanged. Thus, in the words of the Evidence-Based Medicine Working Group (EBMWG), evidence-based practice 'de-emphasizes intuition, unsystematic clinical experience, and pathophysiologic rationale as sufficient grounds for clinical decision making and stresses the examination of *evidence from clinical research*'.[19] As other advocates of evidence-based practice have observed, 'the use of evidence in medicine is certainly not new',[20] but in shifting the rhetoric from 'research' to 'evidence' as the basis for practice, advocates of evidence-based practice have also shifted the definition of what counts as evidence; indeed, they have redefined the word. Thus, 'what *has* changed in clinical medicine in recent decades is the very nature of clinical evidence itself',[21] such that 'case reports have yielded to population-derived studies, of which the randomized controlled trial is the prototype or "gold standard" of therapeutic evidence'.[22] The language has changed, but the sentiments behind it remain the same.

It might, however, be pointed out that things *are* changing, especially in nursing, such that the latest version of evidence-based practice 'is about integrating research evidence with clinical expertise, the resources available and the views of patients'.[23] This statement, made in the first paragraph of a position paper on evidence-based nursing by the Professor of Nursing Research to the DoH, was followed in the second paragraph by the observation that 'in order to deliver evidence-based health care, nurses, like everyone else, need access to high-quality, *research-based information*, to be able to appraise that research, and to decide whether it is good enough to put into practice'.[24] Note the shift from a broad definition of evidence in the first paragraph, which includes clinical expertise, other resources and the views of patients (and which were never again mentioned in the remainder of the paper), to a return to the rhetoric of 'research-based information' in the second. In the very same week, another paper by the Director of Research at the University of Sheffield and some of his colleagues, entitled 'Evidence-based care: can we overcome the barriers?', was taken up entirely with a discussion of how to overcome the barriers to *research*-based care, the word 'evidence' never again appearing after the second paragraph.[25] These are just two examples from many, which happened to be published in the week of writing this epilogue, in which influential writers appear to be embracing a wider definition of evidence-based practice, but are in fact perpetuating the government's covert agenda of attempting to control the discipline of nursing by dictating what counts as the kind of knowledge on which practice should be based. In fact, it is widely recognized that there remains a clear and explicit hierarchy of evidence,[26] such that 'the best evidence is thought to be that obtained from controlled experimental work, and the least value is attached to the authority and clinical experience of the practitioner'.[27]

In contrast to this view, the postmodernist notion of evidence-based practice is much broader, including as evidence not only traditional quantitative research findings (which are stripped of their privileged status and are looked upon with the same incredulity as are all other sources of evidence), but also the extensive and diverse range of qualitative methodologies, other forms of research, experiential knowledge, narrative accounts from other practitioners and from patients, extracts from novels, poetry and film, in fact a complete range of life experiences from within and outside nursing. Furthermore, for the postmodernist nurse, evidence-based practice means not only practice that is *determined* by evidence, but also practice that is *justified* by evidence. In other words, it is not necessary for the evidence to be present at the time when a plan of action is formulated. The nurse might well act according to her intuitive understanding of the clinical situation, and only afterwards justify her actions by reflecting on her practice, thereby producing evidence to support it.

As we have seen, however, from within the modernist discourse of Project 2000 nursing, very little of the above qualifies as evidence, and hence it cannot (by definition) produce good evidence-based practice. However, the postmodernist is not concerned with defending or justifying such practice, which is in any case impossible from within the dominant modernist discourse, but with pointing out that postmodernist practice *cannot* be justified outside the discourse of postmodernism, just as modernist practice cannot be justified from outside the discourse of modernism. By uncovering the hidden power-games being played out in nursing, the aim of the postmodernist is to point out that there is nothing intrinsic to the nature of the randomized controlled trial that make it suitable as evidence, and nothing intrinsic to the nature of reflection-on-action, or even of poetry, that makes it unsuitable.

The postmodernist Project 2001 nurse therefore views *all* paradigms, *all* discourses, *all* models of practice ironically; that is, she regards them all as little narratives, as partial accounts without any absolute claim on the truth. Nursing in this swampy lowland of practice, with no certainty and no guarantee of a successful outcome, brings with it both advantages and disadvantages. On the one hand, the Project 2001 nurse lacks the absolute conviction of her modernist colleagues; she has no gold standard on which to base her practice or on which to justify it afterwards. On the other hand, however, she is not bound by the rigours and restrictions of one particular paradigm, or by the expectation that any one paradigm will always deliver the most appropriate solution to her clinical problems. As we have seen, it is not the case for the postmodernists that anything goes, but instead that nothing is ruled out. From her ironist perspective, the Project 2001 nurse can play whatever (language) game is most appropriate at the time in the full realization that it is, after all, just a game with a more or less arbitrary set of rules. She might, for example, write poetry as a way of coming to understand her own practice, while at the same time submitting a proposal for funding to conduct a strict randomized controlled trial. Or she might bend the rules of survey methodology by including her own reflective and reflexive observations (what positivist researchers refer to disparagingly as 'method slurring').There is, as far as she is concerned, nothing contradictory in any of this: all are simply local solutions to local problems, and none is taken too seriously by being overinvested with credibility.

A memorable fancy

As the title of this book suggests, its aim has been to explore the links between the three concepts of research, truth and authority. I hope I have shown that they form a rather incestuous *menage à trois* in which a few people (hardly ever practitioners) are invested with the power and authority to define what counts as research and how it is to be conducted, which in turn determines what constitutes knowledge and truth, and which ultimately reinforces the authority of those in power and the power of those in authority. Most challenges to this dominant modernist paradigm can be dealt with through the covert imposition of power; so, for example, the qualitative research paradigm is being starved out through lack of funding and written out as non-funded, small-scale project work, and hence, not 'real' research. However, postmodernism is different insofar as it seeks to uncover the very power strategies through which it is being persecuted; it is attempting not to compete with modernism, but to demonstrate the ways in which the modernist discourse has made it *impossible* to compete.

Thus, in answer to the question 'Why not postmodernism?' asked at the beginning of this epilogue, it appears to me that postmodernism poses a particularly acute threat to the modernist discourse of nursing that cannot be dealt with through the usual means, since its aim is precisely to reveal the 'usual means' for what they really are: the imposition of power in the guise of academic rationality. All that is left, then, is to ridicule postmodernism, to label it (as did Melanie Philips, cited in the preface) as 'nihilistic, politically correct gibberish'. This also accounts for the inflated claims made for Socal and Bricmont's book *Intellectual Impostures* (see Chapter 2) as a demonstration that 'modern French philosophy is a load of old tosh', and as 'a devastating critique of some of France's best-known thinkers', when it was clearly nothing of the sort.

William Blake, that first postmodernist, related an allegorical 'Memorable Fancy' in which:

> An angel came to me and said: 'O pitiable foolish young man! O horrible! O dreadful state! consider the hot burning dungeon thou art preparing for thyself to all eternity, to which thou art going in such a career'.[28]

The angel then proceeded to take him on a guided tour of the full horrors of Hell. However, after the angel had gone, Blake tells us, 'I remain'd alone, and then this appearance was no more, but I found myself sitting on a pleasant bank beside a river by moonlight, hearing a harper who sung to the harp'.[29] Blake then rejoined the angel, who was surprised and asked how he had escaped from Hell. 'I answer'd: "All that we saw was owing to your metaphysics; for when you ran away, I found myself on a bank by moonlight hearing a harper. But now we have seen my eternal lot, shall I shew you yours?"'[30] Blake then took the angel on a tour of the heavens, which included some rather blasphemous references to the Christian religion. He concluded his 'memorable fancy' thus:

> So the Angel said: 'thy phantasy has imposed upon me and thou oughtest to be ashamed'. I answer'd: 'we impose on one another, and it is but lost time to converse with you whose works are only Analytics'.[31]

From within *any* belief system or paradigm, what we see is owing to the metaphysics of that paradigm: we see a poem as beautiful largely because of the metaphysics of a particular literary tradition; we see the findings of a randomized controlled trial as true because of the metaphysics of the scientific tradition. As Blake said, over two hundred years ago, we impose on one another, and most disputes between subscribers to different metaphysical systems are merely lost time. Most writers begin optimistically with the intention of rebutting their critics and of demonstrating the superiority of their particular metaphysics. As an eighth-century monk put it, 'it is more valuable to write books than to plant vines, since he who plants a vine feeds his stomach, while he who writes a book feeds his soul'.[32] The postmodernist writer, however, sees behind the truth claims of particular metaphysical systems and the futility of arguments between competing paradigms. In the end, to quote another monk and scholar, 'like the sailor arriving at the port, so the writer rejoices on arriving at the last line. *De gratias semper*'.[33] There is nothing more to be said.

NOTES

1. Blake, W. *The Marriage of Heaven and Hell*, 1793.
2. Bines, H. Issues in course design. In H. Bines & D. Watson (eds) *Developing Professional Education*, Buckingham: Open University Press, 1992. We might also say that it was a move from pre-modernist to modernist nursing.
3. Schön, D. *The Reflective Practitioner*, New York: Basic Books, 1983. Schön, D. *Educating the Reflective Practitioner*, San Francisco: Jossey-Bass, 1987.
4. Schön, D., *op. cit.*, 1987, p. 8.
5. *Ibid.*, p. 3.

6. See, for example, Cook, S. Mind the theory/practice gap in nursing, *Journal of Advanced Nursing*, 1991, **16**, 1462-9; and also Lindsay, B. The gap between theory and practice, *Nursing Standard*, 1990, **5**, 4, 34–5, who states that the theory–practice gap is 'an indication of growth' (p. 34).

7. Rafferty, A.M., Allcock, N. and Lathlean, J. The theory/practice 'gap': taking issue with the issue, *Journal of Advanced Nursing*, 1996, **23**, 685-91. It is difficult to imagine a similar argument being applied in other disciplines. Consider, for example, a civil engineer saying that she is sorry that a bridge has just collapsed, but that it is necessary to maintain a gap between what we know in theory and what we do in practice.

8. You might object that the new millennium started in the year 2000, so Project 2000 has the rightful claim to being the definitive nursing model for the new millennium (and this was clearly part of the reasoning behind its title). However, it has been pointed out that since the first millennium started in the year 1 (there being no year 0), the second millennium started in the year 1001, and the third in the year 2001. This reasoning consigns Project 2000 to the last gasps of a dying technocratic philosophy, and Project 2001 to a new post-technocratic world-view.

9. A full discussion of this argument is presented in Chapter 3.

10. For example, the British government's assertion, based on so-called 'scientific' evidence, that genetically modified (GM) foods are safe, is a political decision disguised as a scientific one. There can, at this early stage, be no scientific evidence that GM foods are safe, but only a lack of evidence that they are harmful.

11. Lyotard, J.-F. (1983) *The Differend: Phrases in Dispute*, G. Van Den Abeele (trans.), Minneapolis: University of Minnesota Press, 1998, p. 142.

12. Marks-Maran, D. Reconstructing nursing: evidence, artistry and the curriculum, *Nurse Education Today*, 1999, **19**, 3–11.

13. Department of Health. *Report of the Taskforce on the Strategy for Research in Nursing, Midwifery and Health Visiting*, London: DoH, 1993, p. 6, emphasis added.

14. *Ibid.*, p. 6.

15. *Ibid.*, p. 6.

16. *Ibid.*, p. 6.

17. *Ibid.*, p. 6.

18. Benner, for example, regarded it as novice practice.

19. Evidence-Based Medicine Working Group. Evidence-based medicine: a new approach to teaching the practice of medicine, *Journal of the American Medical Association*, 1992, **268**, 17, 2420–5, p. 2420, emphasis added.

20. Davidoff, F., Case, K. and Fried, P.W. Evidence-based medicine: why all the fuss?, *Annals of Internal Medicine*, 1995, **122**, 9, 727.

21. *Ibid.*, p. 727.

22. *Ibid.*, p. 727. Davidoff *et al.* have not only redefined the word 'evidence' as being more or less synonymous with the findings from randomized

controlled trials, but have redefined 'prototype' (a trial model or preliminary version) as 'gold standard'.

23. Thompson, D. Why evidence-based nursing, *Nursing Standard*, 1998, **13**, 9, 58–9.

24. *Ibid.*, p. 58.

25. Nolan, M., Morgan, L., Curran, M., Clayton, J., Gerrish, K. and Parker K. Evidence-based care: can we overcome the barriers? *British Journal of Nursing*, 1988, **7**, 20, 1273–8.

26. Rosenberg, W. and Donald, A. Evidence based medicine: an approach to clinical problem-solving, *British Journal of Medicine*, 1995, **310**, 1122–6.

27. White, S.J. Evidence-based practice and nursing: the new panacea? *British Journal of Nursing*, 1997, **6**, 3, 175–8.

28. Blake, W. (1793) The Marriage of Heaven and Hell. In M. Plowman (ed.) *Poems and Prophesies*, London: Dent, 1970, p. 50.

29. *Ibid.*, p. 51. He pointedly continued: 'and his theme was "The man who never alters his opinion is like standing water, & breeds reptiles of the mind"'.

30. *Ibid.*, p. 51.

31. *Ibid.*, p. 52.

32. Alcuin, an eighth-century English monk.

33. Anonymous, twelfth-century monk.

BIBLIOGRAPHY

Then I asked: 'does a firm perswasion that a thing is so, make it so?'
He replied: 'All poets believe that it does,
& in ages of imagination this firm perswasion removed mountains'[1]

Alasuutari, P. *Researching Culture*, London: Sage, 1995.

American Association of Critical Care Nurses *A Model for Differentiated Nursing Practice*, Washington: AACN Press, 1995.

Anderton, W.T. *The Fontana Postmodernism Reader*, London: Fontana, 1996.

Assiter, A. *Enlightened Women: Modernist Feminism in a Postmodern Age*, London: Routledge, 1996.

Bacon, F. *The New Organon and Related Writings*, F.H. Anderson (ed.), New York: Macmillan, 1985.

Bacon, F. *The Great Instauration*, J. Weinberger (ed.) J. Spedding (trans.), Arlington Heights, IL: Harlan Davidson, 1989.

Ball, S. *Politics and Policy Making in Education: Explorations in Policy Sociology*, London: Routledge, 1990.

Barrett, M. and Phillips, A. *Destabilizing Theory: Contemporary Feminist Debates*, Cambridge: Polity Press, 1992.

Barry, P. *Beginning Theory*, Manchester: Manchester University Press, 1995.

Barthes, R. To write: an intransitive verb. In R. Macksey and E. Donato (eds) *The Language of Criticism and the Sciences of Man*, Baltimore: John Hopkins University Press, 1970.

Barthes, R. *The Pleasure of the Text*, New York: Hill & Wang, 1971.

Barthes, R. *Mythologies*, New York: Hill & Wang, 1972.

Barthes, R. *S/Z*, London: Cape, 1975.

Barthes, R. Introduction to the structural analysis of narratives. In R. Barthes *Image Music Text*, S. Heath (trans.), London: Fontana, 1977.

Barthes, R. The death of the author. In R. Barthes *Image Music Text*, S. Heath (trans.), London: Fontana, 1977.

Barthes, R. Writers, intellectuals, teachers. In R. Barthes *Image Music Text*, London: Fontana, 1977.

Barthes, R. *Image Music Text*, London: Fontana, 1977.

Barthes, R. *A Lover's Discourse*, New York: Hill & Wang, 1984.

Barthes, R. *Roland Barthes by Roland Barthes*, London: Macmillan, 1995.

Bateson, G. *Steps to an Ecology of Mind*, New York: Ballantine, 1972.

Baudrillard, J. *Simulations*, New York: Semiotext(e), 1983.

Baudrillard, J. The precession of simulacra. In B. Wallis (ed.) *After Modernism: Rethinking Representation*, Boston: David Godive Publishing, 1984.

Bauman, Z. *Modernity and Ambivalence*, Cambridge: Polity Press, 1991.

Becker, H.S. *Writing for Social Scientists*, Chicago: University of Chicago Press, 1986.

Benner, P. *From Novice to Expert*, Menlo Park, CA: Addison-Wesley, 1984.

Bernstein, R. *Beyond Objectivism and Relativism*, Oxford: Basil Blackwell, 1983.

Bhaskar, R. *The Possibility of Naturalism: A Critique of the Contemporary Human Sciences*, Brighton: Harvester, 1979.

Bhaskar, R. Realism in the natural sciences. In R. Bhaskar *Reclaiming Reality*, London: Verso, 1989.

Bhaskar, R. What is critical realism? In R. Bhaskar *Reclaiming Reality*, London: Verso, 1989.

Billig, M. Sod Baudrillard! Or ideology critique in Disney world. In H.W. Simons and M. Billig (eds) *After Postmodernism: Reconstructing Ideology Critique*, London: Sage, 1994.

Bines, H. Issues in course design. In H. Bines and D. Watson (eds) *Developing Professional Education*, Buckingham: Open University Press, 1992.

Blackburn, S. *The Oxford Dictionary of Philosophy*, Oxford: Oxford University Press, 1994.

Blake, W. The Marriage of Heaven and Hell. In M. Plowman (ed.) *Poems and Prophesies*, London: Dent, 1970.

Blum, A. *Theorising*, London: Heinemann Educational, 1974.

Bohm, D. and Hiley, B. On the intuitive understanding of nonlocality as implied by quantum theory, *Foundations of Physics*, Volume 5, 1975.

Bohr, N. *Atomic Physics and the Description of Nature*, London: Cambridge University Press, 1934.

Bordo, S. Feminism, postmodernism and gender scepticism. In L.J. Nicholson (ed.) *Feminism/Postmodernism*, London: Routledge, 1990.

Borges, J.L. *Labyrinths*, Harmondsworth: Penguin, 1981.

Boyne, R. and Rattsini, A. (eds) *Postmodernism and Society*, London: Macmillan, 1990.

Briggs, J. and Peat, D. *Turbulent Mirror: An Illustrated Guide to Chaos Theory and the Science of Wholeness*, New York: Harper & Row, 1989.

Britzman, D.P. *Practice Makes Practice: A Critical Study of Learning to Teach*, Albany: State University of New York Press, 1991.

Brown, R.H. Reconstructing social theory after the postmodern critique. In H.W. Simons and M. Billig (eds) *After Postmodernism: Reconstructing Ideology Critique*, London: Sage, 1994.

Buckle, H.T. *History of Civilization in England*, Volume 1, London: Longmans, 1861.

Burnard, P. Writing for publication: a guide for those who must, *Nurse Education Today*, 1995, **15**, 117–20.

Butler, J. *Gender Trouble, Feminism and the Subversion of Identity*, London: Routledge, 1990.

Butler, J. Contingent foundations: feminism and the question of 'postmodernism'. In J. Butler and J.W. Scott (eds) *Feminists Theorise the Political*, London: Routledge, 1992.

Butler, J. *Bodies That Matter: The Discursive Limits of 'Sex'*, Routledge: New York, 1993.

Cahoone, L. *From Modernism to Postmodernism: An Anthology*, Malden, MA: Blackwell, 1996.

Carey, J. (ed.) *The Faber Book of Science*, London: Faber and Faber, 1995.

Certeau, M. de *The Practice of Everyday Life*, Berkeley: University of California Press, 1984.

Chambers, I. *Border Dialogues: Journeys in Postmodernity*, London: Routledge, 1990.

Charman, J. *2 Deaths In 1 Night*, Auckland: New Women's Press, 1987.

Chesterton, G.K. *G.F. Watts*, London: Macmillan, 1904, p. 88.

Clarke, L. The last post? Defending nursing against the postmodernist maze, *Journal of Psychiatric and Mental Health Nursing*, 1996, **3**, 257–65.

Clifford, J. *The Predicament of Culture: Twentieth Century Ethnography, Literature and Art*, Cambridge, MA: Harvard University Press, 1988.

Clifford, J. and Marcus, G.E. *Writing Culture: The Poetics and Politics of Ethnography*, Berkeley: University of California Press, 1986.

Closs, S.J. and Draper, P. Commentary, *Nurse Education Today*, 1998, **18**, 337–41.

Condorcet, Marquis de. *Sketch for a Historical Picture of the Progress of the Human Mind*, S. Hampshire (ed.), J. Barraclough (trans.), London: Weidenfeld & Nicolson, 1955.

Cook, S. Mind the theory/practice gap in nursing, *Journal of Advanced Nursing*, 1991, **16**, 1462–9.

Cranston, M. *Philosophers and Pamphleteers*, Oxford: Oxford University Press, 1985.

Dancy, J. and Sosa, E. *A Companion to Epistemology*, Oxford: Blackwell, 1992.

Davidoff, F., Case, K. and Fried, P.W. Evidence-based medicine: why all the fuss? *Annals of Internal Medicine*, 1995, **122**, 9, 727.

De Concini, B. *Narrative Remembering*, Lanham: University of America Press, 1990.

Denzin, N.K. *Interpretive Ethnography*, London: Sage, 1997.

Denzin, N. and Lincoln, Y. *Handbook of Qualitative Research*, Menlo Park, CA: Sage, 1994.

Department of Health. *Report of the Taskforce on the Strategy for Research in Nursing, Midwifery and Health Visiting*, London: DoH, 1993.

Department of Health. *The Nursing and Therapy Professions' Contribution to Health Services Research and Development*. London: DoH, 1995.

Derrida, J. *Of Grammatology*, G.C. Spivak (trans.), Baltimore: John Hopkins University Press, 1974.

Derrida, J. *The Post Card*, Chicago: University of Chicago Press, 1987.

Derrida, J. *Glas*, Lincoln: University of Nebraska Press, 1990.

Docherty, T. *Postmodernism: A Reader*, New York: Harvester Wheatsheaf, 1993.

Dowd, M. *Earthspirit: A Handbook for Nurturing an Ecological Christianity*, Mystic, CT: Twenty Third Publications, 1991.

Dowling, W.C. *Jameson, Althusser, Marx: An Introduction to the Political Unconsciousness*, Ithica, NY: Cornell University Press, 1984.

Durkheim, E. *Suicide: A Study in Sociology*, London: Routledge & Kegan Paul, 1952.

Durkheim, E. *The Rules of Sociological Method*, G. Catlin (ed.), New York: Free Press, 1966.

Eagleton, T. *Literary Theory*, Oxford: Blackwell, 1983.

Ebbutt, D. Educational action research: some general concerns and specific quibbles. In R.G. Burgess (ed.) *Issues in Educational Research: Qualitative Methods*, Lewes: Falmer Press, 1985.

Ebert, T. Review of '*Feminism/Postmodernism*', *Women's Review of Books*, 1991, **8**, 4, 24–5.

Elliott, J. *Action Research for Educational Change*, Milton Keynes, Open University Press, 1991.

Ellis C. and Bochner A.P. *Composing Ethnography*, Walnut Creek: AltaMira, 1996.

Evidence-Based Medicine Working Group. Evidence-based medicine: a new approach to teaching the practice of medicine, *Journal of the American Medical Association*, 1992, **268**, 17, 2420–5.

Féral, J. The powers of difference. In H. Eisenstein and A. Jardine (eds) *The Future of Difference*, New Brunswick: Rutgers University Press, 1980.

Fernández-Armesto, F. *Truth: A History*, London: Bantam Press, 1997.

Ferrucci, P. *What We May Be*, New York: St Martins Press, 1982.

Feyerabend, P.K. Explanation, reduction, and empiricism. In H. Feigl and G. Maxwell (eds) *Scientific Explanation, Space, and Time: Minnesota Studies in the Philosophy of Science*, Volume 3, Minneapolis: University of Minnesota Press, 1962.

Feyerabend, P.K. *Against Method*, London: Verso, 1975.

Feyerabend, P.K. *Against Method*, 3rd edn, London: Verso, 1993.

Field, P.A. and Morse, J.M. *Nursing Research: The Application of Qualitative Approaches*, London: Chapman & Hall, 1985.

Fielding Institute. Research Methodologies, unpublished report, Santa Barbara, CA, 1992.

Fine, M. Passions, politics and power: feminist research possibilities. In M. Fine (ed.) *Disruptive Voices*, Ann Arbor, MI: University of Michigan Press, 1992.

Firestone, S. *The Dialectic of Sex*, New York: Bantam, 1970.

Flax, J. Postmodernism and gender relations in feminist theory, *Signs*, 1978, **8**, 2, 202–23.

Flax, J. Gender as a social problem: in and for feminist theory, *Journal of the German Association for American Studies*, 1986.

Flax, J. *Thinking Fragments: Psychoanalysis, Feminism and Postmodernism in the Contemporary West*, Berkeley: University of California Press, 1990.

Flax, J. The end of innocence. In J. Butler and J.W. Scott (eds) *Feminists Theorise the Political*, London: Routledge, 1992.

Ford-Gilboe, M., Campbell, J. and Berman, H. Stories and numbers: coexistence without compromise, *Advances in Nursing Science*, 1995, **18**, 1, 14–26.

Foucault, M. *The Order of Things: An Archaeology of the Human Sciences*, London: Tavistock, 1974.

Foucault, M. *The Archaeology of Knowledge*, London: Tavistock, 1974.

Foucault, M. *Discipline and Punish: The Birth of the Prison*, New York: Pantheon, 1977.

Foucault, M. *The History of Sexuality*, Volume 1: *An Introduction*, London: Allen Lane, 1979.

Foucault, M. *Power/Knowledge: Selected Interviews and Other Writings 1972–77*, Brighton: Harvester, 1980.

Foucault, M. Introduction. In P. Rabinow (ed.) *The Foucault Reader: An Introduction to Foucault's Thought*, New York: Pantheon Books, 1984.

Fowler, W.S. *The Development of Scientific Method*, Oxford: Pergamon Press, 1962.

Fraser, N. and Nicholson, L. Social criticism without philosophy: an encounter between feminism and postmodernism. In A. Ross (ed.) *Universal Abandon? The Politics of Postmodernism*, Edinburgh: Edinburgh University Press, 1988.

Gadamer, H.-G. *The Enigma of Health*, Cambridge: Polity Press, 1996.

Galileo. *Dialogue Concerning Two Chief World Systems*, 2nd rev. edn, S. Drake (trans.), California: University of California Press, 1967.

Garcia, A.M. The development of Chicana feminist discourse 1970–1980, *Gender and Society*, 1989, **3**, 2, 217–38.

Geertz, C. *The Interpretation of Culture*, New York: Basic Books, 1973.

Geertz, C. *Works and Lives: The Anthropologist as Author*, Stanford, CT: Stanford University Press, 1988.

Giddens, A. *Sociology*, Cambridge: Polity Press, 1989.

Giddens, A. *The Consequences of Modernity*, Cambridge: Polity Press, 1990.

Gill, R. Relativism, reflexivity and politics: interrogating discourse analysis from a feminist perspective. In S. Wilkinson and C. Kitzinger, *Feminism and Discourse: Psychological Perspectives*, London: Sage, 1995.

Giroux, H. Introduction. In P. Freire *The Politics of Education: Culture, Power and Liberation*, D. Macedo (trans.) Basingstoke: Macmillan, 1985.

Gitlin, T. Postmodernism: roots and politics. In I. Angus and S. Ghally (eds), *Cultural Politics in Contemporary America*, Routledge: London, 1989.

Gleick, J. *Chaos: Making a New Science*, London: Cardinal, 1988.

Gower, B. *Scientific Method*, London: Routledge, 1997.

Green, R. The Pocohontas perplex: the image of Indian women in American culture. In E. Dubois and V.L. Ruiz (eds) *Unequal Sisters: A Multi-cultural Reader in US Women's History*, Calgary: Detselig, 1990.

Grosz, E. *Sexual Subversions: Three French Feminists*, North Sydney: Allen & Unwin, 1989.

Grosz, E. *Jacques Lacan: A Feminist Introduction*, London: Routledge, 1990.

Haack, S. Entry on Peirce. In J. Dancy and E. Sosa (eds) *A Companion to Epistemology*, Oxford: Blackwell, 1993.

Habermas, J. Modernity – an incomplete project, *New German Critique*, 1981, **22**, 3–15.

Habermas, J. *The Theory of Communicative Action – Lifeworld and System: A Critique of Functionalist Reason*, Volume 2, Cambridge: Polity Press, 1987.

Habermas, J. *Postmetaphysical Thinking: Philosophical Essays*, Cambridge: MIT Press, 1992.

Hall, S. The toad in the garden: Thatcherism among the theorists. In C. Nelson and L. Grossberg (eds), *Marxism and the Interpretation of Culture*, London: Macmillan, 1988.

Hamilton, E. and Cairns, H. *The Collected Dialogues of Plato*, Princeton, NJ: Princeton University, 1961.

Hamlyn, D.W. *A History of Western Philosophy*, Harmondsworth: Penguin, 1987.

Hammersley, M. and Atkinson, P. *Ethnography: Principles in Practice*, London: Routledge, 1983.

Harding, S. *Feminism and Methodology: Social Science Issues*, Milton Keynes: Open University Press, 1987.

Harding, S. Conclusion: Epistemological questions. In S. Harding (ed.) *Feminism and Methodology: Social Science Issues*, Bloomington: Indiana University Press, 1987.

Harding, S. Is there a feminist method? In N. Tuana (ed.) *Feminism and Science*, Bloomington: Indiana University Press, 1989.

Harding, S. *Whose Science? Whose Knowledge? Thinking from Women's Lives*, Oxford: Oxford University Press, 1991.

Hartsock, N. Foucault on power: a theory for women? In L. Nicholson (ed.) *Feminism/Postmodernism*, New York: Routledge, 1990.

Hassan, I. POSTmodernISM: a paracritical bibliography. In L. Cahoone (ed.) *From Modernism to Postmodernism: An Anthology*, Oxford: Blackwell, 1996.

Hawkesworth, M. Knowers, knowing, known: feminist theory and claims of truth. In M.R. Malson, J.F. O'Barr, W. Westphal and M. Wyer (eds), *Feminist Theory in Practice and Process*, Chicago: University of Chicago Press, 1989.

Hayman, R. *Nietzsche*, London: Phoenix, 1997.

Heidegger, M. *Being and Time*, J. Macquarie and E. Robinson (trans.) Oxford: Basil Blackwell, 1962.

Heidegger, M. *Poetry, Language, Thought*, A. Hofstadter (trans.), New York: Harper & Row, 1971.

Heisenberg, W. *Physics and Philosophy*, London: Allen & Unwin, 1963.

Heller, A. and Feher, F. *The Postmodern Political Condition*, Cambridge: Polity Press, 1988.

Heller, A. and Feher, F. *The Grandeur and Twilight of Radical Universalism*, New Jersey: Transaction Publishers, 1991.

Henley, J. Euclidean, Spinozist or existentialist? Er, no. It's simply a load of old tosh, *Guardian*, 1 October, 1997, p. 3.

Hill Collins, P. *Black Feminist Thought: Knowledge, Consciousness, and the Politics of Empowerment*, Boston: Unwin Hyman, 1990.

Hillis-Miller, J. Narrative. In F. Lentdcchia and T. McLaughlin (eds) *Critical Terms for Literary Study*, Chicago: University of Chicago Press, 1990.

Hollis, M. *The Philosophy of Social Science*, Cambridge: Cambridge University Press, 1994.

Holly, M.L. Reflective writing and the spirit of inquiry, *Cambridge Journal of Education*, 1989, **19**, 1, 71–80.

Holmes, C. Critical Theory and the Discourse of Nursing Ethics, unpublished doctoral dissertation, Geelong: Deakin University. 1993.

hooks, b. Choosing the margin as a space of radical openness. In *Yearning: Race, Gender, and Cultural Politics*, Boston, MA: South End Press, 1990.

Horgan, J. *The End of Science: Facing the Limits of Knowledge in the Twilight of the Scientific Age*, London: Abacus, 1996.

Hughes, J. *The Philosophy of Social Research*, London: Longman, 1990.

Hume, D. *Enquiry Concerning Human Understanding*, London: Longman, 1875.

Irigaray, L. *The Sex Which Is Not One*, Ithica, NY: Cornell University Press, 1985.

Jackson, S. The amazing deconstructing woman, *Trouble and Strife*, 1992, **25**, 25–31.

James, W. *Pragmatism*, London: Longman, 1907.

Jameson, F. Postmodernism, or the cultural logic of capital, *New Left Review*, 1984, **146**, 53–92.

Jenkins, K. *Re-thinking History*, London: Routledge, 1991.

Johnson, B. *The Critical Difference*, Baltimore: John Hopkins University Press, 1980.

Johnson, P. *Feminism as Radical Humanism*, St Leonards, NSW: Allen & Unwin, 1994.

Jung, C.G. *On the Nature of the Psyche*, Princeton: Princeton University Press, 1960.

Kant, I. *The Critique of Pure Reason*, N. Kemp Smith (trans.), London: St Martin's Press, 1978.

Katz, S. How to speak and write postmodern. In W.T. Anderson, *The Fontana Postmodernism Reader*, London: Fontana Press, 1996.

Kearney, R. *Modern Movements in European Philosophy*, 2nd edn, Manchester: Manchester University Press, 1994.

Kermode, S. and Brown, C. The postmodernist hoax and its effect on nursing, *International Journal of Nursing Studies*, 1996, **33**, 4, 375–84.

Kincheloe, J.L. and McLaren, P.L. Rethinking critical theory and qualitative research. In N.K. Denzin and Y.S. Lincoln (eds) *Handbook of Qualitative Research*, Thousand Oaks, CA: Sage, 1994.

Kipnis, L. Feminism: the political conscience of postmodernism? In A. Ross (ed.) *Universal Abandon: The Politics of Postmodernism*, Minneapolis: University of Minnesota Press, 1988.

Koestler, A. *The Ghost in the Machine*, London: Pan, 1971.

Komarovsky, M. The new feminist scholarship: some precursors and polemics, *Journal of Marriage and the Family*, 1988, **50**, 585–93.

Kristeva, J. *Desire in Language: A Semiotic Approach to Art and Literature*, L.S. Roudiez (trans.) New York: University of Columbia Press, 1980.

Kritek, P. Negotiating at the Uneven Table, paper presented at Center for Nursing Leadership, Hill-Rom Farm, Batesville, Indiana, 1995.

Kritzman, L.D. (ed.) *Michel Foucault: Politics, Philosophy, Culture. Interviews and Other Writings, 1977–84*, A. Sheridan (trans.), London: Routledge, 1988.

Kuhn, T.S. *The Structure of Scientific Revolutions*, Chicago: University of Chicago Press, 1962.

Kuhn, T.S. Reflections on my critics. In I. Lakatos and A. Musgrave (eds) *Criticism and the Growth of Knowledge*, Cambridge: Cambridge University Press, 1970.

Lamb, G.S. and Stempel, J.E. Nursing case management from the client's view: growing as insider-expert, *Nursing Outlook*, 1994, **42**, 1, 7–13.

Lather, P. *Getting Smart... Feminist Research and Pedagogy With/In the Postmodern*, London: Routledge, 1991.

Lather, P. The Politics and Ethics of Feminist Research: Researching the Lives of Women with AIDS, draft of an address prepared for the Ethnography and Education Research Forum, Philadelphia, PA, 1993.

Lather, P. Staying dumb? Feminist research and pedagogy with/in the postmodern. In H.W. Simons and M. Billig (eds) *After Postmodernism: Reconstructing Ideology Critique*, London: Sage, 1994.

Lawler, J. *Behind the Screens: Nursing, Somatology and the Problem of the Body*, Melbourne: Churchill Livingstone, 1991.

Lindsay, B. The gap between theory and practice, *Nursing Standard*, 1990, **5**, 4, 34–5.

Locke, J. *Essay Concerning Human Understanding*, London: Dent, 1961.

Lorenz, E. Predictability: Does the Flap of a Butterfly's Wings in Brazil set off a Tornado in Texas?, address at the annual meeting of the American Association for the Advancement of Science, Washington, 1979.

Lovibond, S. Feminism and postmodernism. In T. Docherty (ed.) *Postmodernism: A Reader*, New York: Harvester Wheatsheaf, 1993.

Lyotard, J.-F. *The Postmodern Condition: A Report on Knowledge*, Manchester: Manchester University Press, 1984.

Lyotard, J.-F. Answering the question: what is postmodernism? In J.-F. Lyotard *The Postmodern Condition: A Report on Knowledge*, Manchester: Manchester University Press, 1984.

Lyotard, J.-F. Rewriting modernity, *SubStance*, 1987, **54**, 8–9.

Lyotard, J.-F. *The Differend: Phrases in Dispute*, G. Van Den Abbeele (trans.), Minneapolis: University of Minnesota Press, 1988.

Lyotard, J.-F. Apostil on narratives. In J.-F. Lyotard *The Postmodern Explained to Children*, London: Turnaround, 1992.

Lyotard, J.-F. Note on the meaning of 'post-'. In J.-F. Lyotard *The Postmodern Explained to Children*, London: Turnaround, 1992.

Lyotard, J.-F. Ticket for a new stage. In J.-F. Lyotard *The Postmodern Explained to Children*, London: Turnaround, 1992.

Lyotard, J.-F. *The Postmodern Explained to Children*, London: Turnaround, 1992.

Lyotard, J.-F. and Thébaud, J.-L. *Just Gaming*, Minneapolis: University of Minnesota Press, 1979.

McIntyre, M. The focus on the discipline of nursing: a critique and extension, *Advances in Nursing Science*, 1995, **18**, 1, 27–35.

McLaren, P. Schooling the postmodern body: critical pedagogy and the politics of enfleshment, *Journal of Education*, 1988, **170**, 3, 53–83.

McLaren, P. Language, social structure and the production of subjectivity, *Critical Pedagogy Networker*, May/June 1988, **1**, 2, 1–10.

Marcus, G. and Fischer, M. *Anthropology as Cultural Critique: An Experimental Moment in the Human Sciences*, Chicago: University of Chicago Press, 1986.

Marks-Maran, D. Reconstructing nursing: evidence, artistry and the curriculum, *Nurse Education Today*, 1999, **19**, 3–11.

Mehra, J. (ed.) *The Physicist's Conception of Nature*, Dordrecht: Reidel, 1973.

Midgely, M. *Wisdom, Information, and Wonder*, London: Routledge, 1991.

Mill, J.S. *A System of Logic*, 8th edn, London: Longman, 1967.

Mills, C.W. *The Sociological Imagination*, Harmondsworth: Penguin, 1970.

Mitroff, I. *The Scientific Side of Science*, Amsterdam: Elsevier, 1974.

Mohanty, C. Under Western eyes: feminist scholarship and colonial discourses, *Feminist Review*, 1988, **30**, 60–8.

Morse, J.M., *Qualitative Nursing Research: A Contemporary Dialogue*, rev. edn, Newbury Park, CA: Sage, 1991.

Nash, K. The feminist production of knowledge: is deconstruction a practice for women? *Feminist Review*, 1994, **47**, 65–76.

Newman, M. *Health as Expanding Consciousness*, New York: National League for Nursing Press, 1994.

Newman, M.A., Sime, A.M. and Corcoran-Perry, S.A. The focus of the discipline of nursing, *Advances in Nursing Science*, 1991, **14**, 1, 1–6.

Newton, I. *Principia*, Volume 2 (facsimile reprint), A. Motte (trans.), London: Dawsons of Pall Mall, 1968.

Nietzsche, F. *Beyond Good and Evil*, Harmondsworth: Penguin, 1973.

Nietzsche, F. *The Gay Science*, 2nd edn, New York: Random House, 1974.

Nietzsche, F. Human, all too human. In R.J. Hollingdale (ed.) *A Nietzsche Reader*, Harmondsworth: Penguin, 1977.

Nolan, M., Morgan, L., Curran, M., Clayton, J., Gerrish, K. and Parker K. Evidence-based care: can we overcome the barriers? *British Journal of Nursing*, 1988, **7**, 20, 1273–8.

Ornstein, R. *Multimind*, Boston, MA: Houghton Mifflin, 1987.

Parker, J.M. Bodies and boundaries in nursing: a postmodern and feminist analysis, paper delivered at the National Nursing Conference, Science, Reflectivity and Nursing Care: exploring the dialectic. 5–6 December, 1991, Melbourne, Australia.

Parse, R. Human becoming: Parse's theory of nursing, *Nursing Science Quarterly*, 1992, **5**, 1, 35–42.

Parse, R.R. Quality of life: sciencing and living the art of human becoming, *Nursing and Science Quarterly*, 1994, **7**, 1, 16–21.

Pateman, C. *The Sexual Contract*, Cambridge: Polity Press, 1988.

Payne, D. The knives are out for P2000, *Nursing Times*, 1999, **95**, 4, 14–15.

Payne, M. *Reading Theory*, Oxford: Blackwell, 1993.

Peirce, C.S. How to make our ideas clear, *Popular Science Monthly*, 1878, **12**, 286–302.

Phillips, D.L. *Abandoning Method*, London: Jossey-Bass, 1973.

Polit, D.F. and Hungler, B.P. *Nursing Research: Principles and Methods*, 5th edn, Philadelphia: J.B. Lippincott, 1995.

Popper, K.R. *The Logic of Scientific Discovery*, London: Hutchinson, 1959.

Popper, K.R. *Objective Knowledge*, rev. edn, Oxford: Clarendon Press, 1979.

Poster, M. Foucault, the present and history, *Cultural Critique*, 1988, **8**, 105–21.

Putnam, H. *Reason, Truth and History*, Cambridge: Cambridge University Press, 1981.

Quetelet, A. *A Treatise on Man and the Development of his Faculties*, New York: Burt Franklin, 1968.

Quine, W.V.O. Two dogmas of empiricism. In W.V.O. Quine, *From a Logical Point of View*, Cambridge MA: Harvard University Press, 1980.

Rafferty, A.M. *The Politics of Nursing Knowledge*, London: Routledge, 1996.

Rafferty, A.M. Practice made perfect, *Guardian Higher*, 26 January, 1999.

Rafferty, A.M., Allcock, N. and Lathlean, J. The theory/practice 'gap': taking issue with the issue, *Journal of Advanced Nursing*, 1996, **23**, 685–91.

Readings, B. *Introducing Lyotard*, London: Routledge, 1991.

Reason, P. and Rowan, J. *Human Inquiry: A Sourcebook of New Paradigm Research*, Chichester: John Wiley, 1981.

Reinharz, S. *Feminist Methods in Social Research*, New York: Oxford University Press, 1992.

Revill, G. Reading Rosehill community, identity and inner-city Derby. In G. Revill, *Place and the Politics of Identity*, London: Routledge, 1993.

Richardson, L. Writing: a method of inquiry. In N.K. Denzin and Y.S. Lincoln (eds), *Handbook of Qualitative Research*, Thousand Oaks, CA: Sage, 1994.

Ricouer, P. *Hermeneutics and the Human Sciences*, J.B. Thompson (ed.), Cambridge: Cambridge University Press, 1981.

Ricoeur, P. *Lectures on Ideology and Utopia*, G.H. Taylor (ed.), New York: Columbia University Press, 1986.

Rogers, M.E. Science of unitary human beings. In V.M. Malinski (ed.) *Explorations on Martha Rogers' Science of Unitary Beings*, Norwalk, CT: Appleton-Century-Crofts, 1986.

Rolfe, G. *Closing the Theory–Practice Gap*, Oxford: Butterworth Heinemann, 1996.

Rorty, R. *Contingency, Irony, and Solidarity*, Cambridge: Cambridge University Press, 1989.

Rorty, R. Solidarity or objectivity. In R. Rorty, *Objectivity, Relativism, and Truth: Philosophical Papers*, Volume 1, Cambridge, Cambridge University Press, 1991.

Rorty, R. *Objectivity, Relativism, and Truth: Philosophical Papers*, Volume 1, Cambridge, Cambridge University Press, 1991.

Rosenberg, W. and Donald, A. Evidence based medicine: an approach to clinical problem-solving, *British Journal of Medicine*, 1995, **310**, 1122–6.

Rousseau, J.J. Fragment inédit d'un essai sur les langues. In *The Social Contract and Discourses*, G.D.H. Cole (trans.), London: Dent, 1913.

Russell, B. *A History of Western Philosophy*, London: Allen & Unwin, 1946.

Salmon, W. *Logic*, Englewood Cliffs, NJ: Prentice Hall, 1963.

Sandywell, B., Silverman, D., Roche, M., Filmer, P. and Phillipson, M. *Problems of Reflexivity and Dialectics in Sociological Inquiry: Language Theorising Difference*, London: Routledge & Kegan Paul, 1975.

Sarup, M. *An Introductory Guide to Post-structuralism and Postmodernism*, New York: Harvester Wheatsheaf, 1988.

Saussure, F. de *Course in General Linguistics*, London: Duckworth, 1983.

Sawicki, J. Identity politics and sexual freedom. In I. Diamond and L. Quinby (eds) *Feminism and Foucault: Reflections on Resistance*, Boston: Northeastern University Press, 1988.

Schatzman, L. and Strauss, A. *Field Research: Strategies for a Natural Sociology*, Englewood Cliffs, NJ: Prentice Hall, 1973.

Schlipp, P.A. *Albert Einstein, Philosopher-Scientist*, Evanston, IL: Tudor, 1948.

Scholes, R. *Textual Power: Literary Theory and the Teaching of English*, New Haven: Yale University Press, 1985.

Schön, D. *The Reflective Practitioner*, New York: Basic Books, 1983.

Schön, D. *Educating the Reflective Practitioner*, San Francisco: Jossey-Bass, 1987.

Schrag, C.O. *Communicative Praxis and the Space of Subjectivity*, Bloomington: Indiana University Press, 1986.

Scruton, R. *Modern Philosophy*, London: Arrow, 1994.

Sharp, L.F. and Priesmeyer, H.R. Tutorial: Chaos theory – a primer for health care, *Quality Management in Health Care*, 1995, **3**, 4, 71–86.

Sheldrake, R. *A New Science of Life*, London: Paladin, 1981.

Siegel, H. *Relativism Refuted: A Critique of Contemporary Epistemological Relativism*, Dordrecht: Reidel, 1987.

Simons, H. *Towards a Science of the Singular*, Norwich: University of East Anglia, 1980.

Simons, H.W. and Billig, M. *After Postmodernism*, London: Sage, 1994.

Smart, B. *Postmodernity*, London: Routledge, 1993.

Smith, R. *The Fontana History of the Human Sciences*, London: Fontana, 1997.

Sokal, A. and Bricmont, J. *Intellectual Impostures*, London: Profile Books, 1998.

Sorell, T. *Scientism: Philosophy and the Infatuation with Science*, London: Routledge, 1991.

Spivak, G.C. Translator's preface. In J. Derrida, *Of Grammatology*, Baltimore: John Hopkins University Press, 1976.

Spivak, G. *In Other Worlds: Essays in Cultural Politics*, London: Routledge, 1988.

Spradley, J. *The Ethnographic Interview*, New York: Holt, Rinehart & Winston, 1979.

Squiers, J. *Principled Positions: Postmodernism and the Rediscovery of Value*, London: Lawrence & Wishart, 1993.

Stanley, L. and Wise, S. *Breaking Out Again: Feminist Ontology and Epistemology*, 2nd edn, London: Routledge, 1993.

Stenhouse, L. Case study and case records: towards a contemporary history of education, *British Educational Research Journal*, 1978, **4**, 2, 21–39.

Stoller, P. and Olkes, C. *In Sorcery's Shadow: A Memoir of Apprenticeship among the Songhay of Niger*, Chicago: University of Chicago Press, 1987.

Street, A. *Inside Nursing: A Critical Ethnography of Nursing*, New York: State University of New York Press, 1992.

Teilhard du Chardin, P. *The Phenomenon of Man*, New York: Harper & Row, 1959.

Thompson, D. Why evidence-based nursing, *Nursing Standard*, 1998, **13**, 9, 58–9.

Turner, V. and Bruner, E.M. *The Anthropology of Experience*, Urbana: University of Illinois Press, 1986.

Tyler, S. *The Unspeakable: Discourse, Dialogue and Rhetoric in the Postmodern World*, Madison: University of Wisconsin Press, 1987.

Usher, R. and Edwards R. *Postmodernism and Education*, London: Routledge, 1994.

Van Maanen, J. *Tales of the Field: On Writing Ethnography*, Chicago: University of Chicago Press, 1988.

Van Manen, M. *Researching Lived Experience*, New York: State University of New York Press, 1990.

Vinci, L. da. *Codex Atlanticus*, unpublished manuscript, *c.* 1490.

Walker, K. On What it Might Mean To Be a Nurse: a Discursive Ethnography, unpublished doctoral dissertation, Melbourne: La Trobe University, 1993.

Walker, K. Confronting reality: nursing, science, and the micro-politics of representation, *Nursing Inquiry*, 1994, **1**, 46–56.

Walker, K. Courting competency: nursing and the politics of performance in practice, *Nursing Inquiry*, 1995, **2**, 90–9.

Walker, K. Crossing borders: bringing nursing practice, teaching and research together into the 21st century, *International Journal of Nursing Practice*, 1995, **1**, 1, 12–17.

Walker, P.M.B. *Chambers Science and Technology Dictionary*, Edinburgh: Chambers, 1991.

Watson, J.B. *Behaviourism*, London: Kegan Paul, 1925.

Watson, J. *Nursing: Human Science and Human Care*, Norwalk, CT: Appleton-Century-Crofts, 1985.

Waugh, P. Postmodern theory: the current debate. In P. Waugh (ed.) *Postmodernism: A Reader*, London: Hodder & Stoughton, 1992.

Weber, M. *The Protestant Ethic and the Spirit of Capitalism*, London: Unwin, 1930.

Weber, M. *Economy and Society*, Volume 1, New York: Bedminster Press, 1968.

Weber, M. Science as vocation. In P. Lassman and I. Velody, *Max Weber's 'Science as Vocation'*, London: Unwin Hyman, 1989.

Weedon, C. *Feminist Practice and Poststructuralist Theory*, Oxford: Basil Blackwell, 1987.

Wheatley, M. *Leadership and the New Science: Learning about Organization from an Orderly Universe*, San Francisco: Berrett-Koehler, 1992.

White, S.J. Evidence-based practice and nursing: the new panacea? *British Journal of Nursing*, 1997, **6**, 3, 175–8.

Winch, P. *The Idea of a Social Science and its Relation to Philosophy*, 2nd edn, London: Routledge, 1990.

Wittgenstein, L. *Philosophical Investigations*, Oxford: Basil Blackwell, 1953.

Wittgenstein, L. *Tractatus Logico-Philosophicus*, D.F. Pears and B.F. McGuiness (trans.), London: Routledge & Kegan Paul, 1961.

Woolf, V. *A Writer's Diary*, Bungay: Triad Granada, 1978.

Yates, L. Postmodernism, feminism and cultural politics, or if master narratives have been discredited, what does Giroux think he is doing? *Discourse*, 1992, **13**, 1, 124.

Yin, R.K. *Case Study Research*, London: Sage, 1994.

NOTE

1. Blake, W. The Marriage of Heaven and Hell, 1793, in M. Plowman (ed.) *Blakes' Poems and Prophesies*, London: Dent, 1927.